THE SAFE BOX OF HEALTH

3 Steps to Heal Yourself

by

Bradley R. Wilde, D.C.

You can heal yourself!

Brad

Notice

The information given here is designed to help you make informed decisions about your health. It is not intended as a substitute for any treatment that may have been prescribed by your doctor. If you suspect that you have a medical problem, we urge you to seek competent medical help.

Wilde Natural Health Publishing
801 Robertson
Worland, WY 82401
www.drwilde.com
1-866-379-4533

ISBN:1460969170
ISBN-13:978-1460969175

Illustrations by Brenda Suko

Printed in the United States of America

*Dedicated to the thousands of
wonderful patients who taught me
that the body truly does heal itself.*

What Others Are Saying About
THE SAFE BOX OF HEALTH
3 Steps to Heal Yourself

I had a number of health issues, including chronic kidney infections, constant neck and lower back pain, and painful menstrual cycles. As I read this book I realized I was literally making myself sick! As I let go of my emotional baggage, my symptoms completely disappeared. I consider it a *must read* for anyone who is serious about taking responsibility for their own health and happiness. - Heather P.

The book *The Safe Box of Health* is incredible! Before reading the book I did not understand what a strong connection there is between our emotions and how our bodies react to the way we feel and believe. I have learned that nutrition plays a major role in not being sick as well. I have learned that we are in charge of our own lives and that we need to be able to take control! Most of all, I find hope from reading Dr. Wilde's book and the courage to start over when I need to, knowing that we do not have to be perfect - just in control and trying to be better! - Trudy L.

After reading *The Safe Box of Health* I decided to use Dr. Wilde's suggestions to see if I could improve my own health. I had been dealing with many sore spots and painful knots in my upper back and nothing seemed to help. I was amazed, the knots and pains disappeared one by one and have never returned. Dr. Wilde's book is amazing and I am grateful to have had the opportunity to read it. - Karen L.

Menopause symptoms at age 24? I was experiencing all of the classic symptoms: hot flashes, irregular periods, night sweats, mood swings, fatigue, memory lapses, dizziness, weight gain, and many others. I went to a variety of doctors, but received no answers until I met Dr. Wilde. After meeting with Dr. Wilde, reading his book and allowing him to teach me a different perspective on the way the body and the brain function together, I was able to completely overcome my symptoms, get off of all prescription and OTC medications, and get on with an energetic and enjoyable life. Now at age 27 I am doing 100% better. - Alicia B.

The Safe Box of Health is an amazing book! Dr. Wilde has covered it all. I moved some of my unsafe things over into the Safe Box, as Dr. Wilde suggested, and a great weight was lifted off my shoulders. I will continue to move things over. He has presented the information for self-healing in a clear, concise, and logical way. - Meela R.

The Safe Box of Health is a book with a simple yet powerful message that instills hope when you read it! The countless stories of real, every day people overcoming their afflictions cannot be overlooked or dismissed as fantasy. I recommend this book for anyone to read. You will not be disappointed! - Allen N.

It is truly amazing what you can do for yourself to heal yourself! Reading *The Safe Box of Health,* and a few sessions with Dr. Wilde has given me invaluable insight and tools to start removing the layers of emotional and physical pain that a lifetime of stresses has laid down. Thank you Dr. Wilde. - Deb S.

The Safe Box of Health is a wonderful book that spoke truth to my heart. So many of us want to be the victim and blame our illness and struggles in life on something or someone, other than ourselves. By addressing the emotional cause of my problems, I have been able to understand what it is I'm doing to create such a life for myself and know what I must do to change it. By applying the principles taught in *The Safe Box of Health*, healing will take place. Thank you Dr. Wilde for this much needed book! - Sherri J.

The principles Dr. Wilde teaches in *The Safe Box of Health* have greatly enhanced my life and the health and well-being of my whole family. These concepts really work. - Toni C.

The Safe Box and Unsafe Box is a very powerful concept. It has helped me, very quickly, to be able to recognize how the experiences I've put into my Unsafe Box through the years have come back to haunt me emotionally and physically. I'm so very grateful for this book that has helped me learn how to take those out and put them into my Safe Box. The difference already in my attitude and health has been incredible to me. Thank you Dr. Wilde for sharing your wisdom. - Adria S.

Because of some major injuries over several years, I began to have life altering panic attacks and health deterioration. I was very unhappy and thought I was going crazy. Physically, I was having muscle cramps every night and my back hurt all the time. I saw my doctor who diagnosed me with asthma and MS. I first saw Dr. Wilde when he lectured to a women's group and for the first time felt hope. What he taught was life altering. In his book, *The Safe Box of Health,* he teaches principles that will change lives. I know because it changed mine. I have energy, I feel hope, my back and leg muscles feel good and I feel whole again. If someone were to read one book on health, I would highly recommend *The Safe Box of Health* by Dr. Bradley R. Wilde. - Stacey W.

I have applied the principles that Dr. Wilde teaches in *The Safe Box of Health.* As I came from a medical "Doctor Fix me" background it has been a challenge, but I can honestly say I am healthier now than I was 28 years ago. - Ruth R.

Because of the things I have learned from this book, I have been able to avoid surgeries and expensive medications. I would and do highly recommend it!! - Terisa B.

I went through a divorce and was very depressed for over 9 months. On the 10th month I came down with Rheumatoid Arthritis. I know I made myself sick through my sadness, guilt, and regrets. Our thoughts and feelings are so connected to our physical bodies, Dr. Wilde is right on. – Rebecca N.

I have suffered with a stiff and painful neck, bad shoulder pain, and unexplained poor health for many years. Through the principles described in *The Safe Box of Health* I have experienced the pain relief I have needed, both physically and mentally. I've come to understand that physical and mental healing are tied together and forgiving of oneself and others is truly healing. - Betty M.

CONTENTS

PART 1: UNDERSTANDING THE CAUSE OF YOUR SYMPTOMS

PART 2: 3 STEPS TO HEAL YOURSELF

INTRODUCTION

Imagine that you are a sixty year old librarian. You retired one year ago and have enjoyed having time to yourself. One day you bent over and picked up your twelve month old grandson. You felt a twinge of pain in your neck and wrist, but didn't think too much of it. It is now nine months later and the problem is getting worse. You decide that you had better do something about it. Your neck is now chronically sore and your wrist hurts all the time. You can't open a jar with your right hand anymore and are worried that you might lose the use of that hand. What do you do? Where do you go?

Suppose you come see me. You know that I am a chiropractor and have had many years of experience treating patients with similar problems. You think that I might know what to do with your neck and wrist to return them to normal. As we talk, you tell me that you enjoy being home, but that you feel guilty that you are not getting as much accomplished as you should. You wish, in a sense, that you had deadlines again to motivate you.

I tell you that I think that your ailments are more than physical, and are likely due to the guilt you feel. You look at me a little surprised since that is not what you expected. I explain that if you relieve yourself of the guilt, you will also relieve yourself of your neck and wrist pain. You decide to give it a try. Within a week, your neck and wrist are back to normal, like they were nine months earlier.

Though this story really didn't happen to you, it did happen to someone like you. If you are looking for answers to health problems, especially chronic ongoing ones, it's likely that a similar story could be written about you.

Most everyone understands that symptoms such as ulcers and high blood pressure can be related to stress. Few people are aware that a knee pain or shoulder pain may also be stress induced, or possibly related to diet. Even fewer know that ulcers, high blood pressure, knee pain and shoulder pain may be due to a memory of a past experience or a feeling that their bodies have been programmed to respond to.

While stress, memories, emotions, or diet are not the cause of all symptoms, they are the instigator of many. In fact, they are much more common causes than we generally suppose. You can easily treat the majority of your symptoms if you understand the **cause**.

Of course there are health care professionals who can answer questions and help with major or serious problems, and you should always consult them. But the more you learn and understand about how your body works, and why it is doing what it is doing, the more you will be able to take charge and heal yourself.

At the conclusion of this book, you should understand the **cause** of your symptoms and know how to fix them. I would hope that when you are done reading, you will know how to heal yourself, just like the librarian.

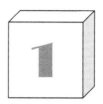

WHY DO I HURT?

Eric (all names have been changed) had a sharp pain in his neck and shoulders. He could hardly turn his head and had severe pain in his right arm. Eric worked as a mechanic. He found it almost impossible to work under any equipment where he had to lift his hands above his head, as that greatly intensified the pain.

Chiropractic treatments helped Eric some, but the relief didn't seem to last very long. I suggested stress could intensify an ailment and Eric volunteered that he was having money problems as well as some problems with his boss.

A few days later Eric came bounding into my office, 90% improved. He had solved his problem. He said he had had a slow time at work and had taken time off to go to the bank to resolve a few bounced checks. When he returned to work his boss blew up at him as he had not given Eric permission to leave. That was more than Eric could take. He threw up his hands and said, *"I quit! I don't need any more of this!"* As he drove home from work, he could feel the tension gradually leaving his neck and shoulders. By the next morning he was almost completely pain free.

Amber told me that if I couldn't help her, she was going to have her foot amputated. She'd had twenty surgeries on her foot in nineteen years, and was just getting out of the boot she had worn since surgery a year earlier. It had all started as a ten year old when she had caught her foot in a merry-go-round. She'd had constant pain in her foot since, and the surgeries hadn't helped relieve the pain. Now she was the mother of a small child and was expecting twins, and didn't know how she could continue the way things were.

I suggested to Amber that something was interfering with the healing message that normally goes from the brain to an injured area of the body, like a short circuit, the most likely cause being some emotional trauma from the time of the injury. She had a few ideas of what they were, and was able to start working on healing those negative emotions. To her amazement, as she was leaving the treatment room, for the first time in several years, she was able to take a few steps without any pain. It was the beginning of a wonderful healing process for her.

Dan's shoulder had been hurting for two months, and wasn't getting any better. It kept him from sleeping at night, and he couldn't get his arm above his head.

We treated Dan a couple of times, but it didn't improve very much. When I asked about his diet, I could see that this might be the source of some of his problems. So I asked him to cut back on his coffee, and add two fruits a day to his diet. In five days he had full range of motion, and was once again sleeping through the night.

The stories of these three individuals are actual case histories and are typical of many others. They all have two things in common:

1. **Each person did not understand the cause of his or her symptoms.**
2. **Each person was able to fix his or her symptoms once he or she understood the cause.**

There is a good chance you are like these people. The purpose of this book is to help you understand the cause of your symptoms so *You Can Heal Yourself.* Physical and emotional trauma, bad memories, fears, worries, stress, and a poor diet affect all of us and eventually lead to unwanted symptoms. The body does not make mistakes! It is acting on the messages it is being given and it responds accordingly, even though we may not like what it is doing. Stress is a natural and essential part of life, yet our reactions to it play a much greater role in poor health than most people realize.

Before you continue, make a list of pain or other physical symptoms you have. Then rate those symptoms on a scale of 1-10, with 10 being the worst. Having these symptoms in mind will help you relate to what you read, and help you better understand the solutions.

SYMPTOMS	SEVERITY
1	1 2 3 4 5 6 7 8 9 10
2	1 2 3 4 5 6 7 8 9 10
3	1 2 3 4 5 6 7 8 9 10
4	1 2 3 4 5 6 7 8 9 10
5	1 2 3 4 5 6 7 8 9 10

There are Two Parts to this book and both are necessary to help you heal yourself and be well.

Part One, Understanding the Cause of Your Symptoms, is to help you understand how your body and mind work together, how poor nutrition affects you, and why physical symptoms become normal and necessary. If you have unresolved health problems, you should gain a great deal of insight to their cause from this section.

Part Two, 3 Steps to Heal Yourself is a 3 Step Guide explaining how to apply lessons learned in Part One. We will summarize and further expound on the steps you can follow to achieve healing and wellness so physical symptoms are no longer normal or necessary.

Both parts of this book are important. As you incorporate these concepts and ideas into your life, you will be absolutely amazed at the healing experience you will have.

Part 1

UNDERSTANDING THE CAUSE OF YOUR SYMPTOMS

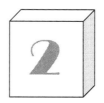

THE SAFE BOX
AND THE UNSAFE BOX

Several years ago, I was asked to speak to a women's group about stress management. To enhance my presentation, I took along our 7 month old daughter, Brittany. As I began the class, I carefully stood Brittany up in my right hand, and balanced her in front of the audience. How do you think these ladies reacted?

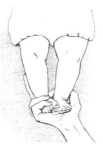

Write down or mentally note what your reactions would be. To make it a little more personal, imagine that I am balancing your baby or grandchild in my hand. Identify what you think your emotions (feelings) would be as well as the changes your physical body (symptoms) would experience.

FEELINGS	SYMPTOMS
1._____	1._____
2._____	2._____
3._____	3._____
4._____	4._____
5._____	5._____

After a few muffled gasps from the women, I asked the president of the group how she reacted to the demonstration. She exclaimed, *"Oh, I'm sweating!"* Other responses followed. *"I was afraid!"* *"I felt anxious!"* One eighty year old lady was very irritated and said, *"I would like to hit people who do that! Suppose that baby fell!"*

We made a list on the chalkboard of reactions that the ladies experienced. Here's the list.

FEELINGS	SYMPTOMS
1. Fear	1. Sweating
2. Anxiety	2. Increased Heart Rate
3. Anger	3. Tense Muscles
4. Worry	4. Nervous Stomach
	5. Held Breath

It was obvious that these women were influenced by this little demonstration.

Now, consider Brittany. What were the feelings and symptoms she experienced? Here is the short list the women wrote down.

FEELINGS	SYMPTOMS
1. Safe	1. Smiling
2. Happy	

The active participant in this experiment was Brittany. She was the one at risk, yet she displayed no sign whatsoever of stress. Meanwhile, every lady in the room was an observer, and yet almost every one of them experienced at least one of the previously mentioned reactions. Why was this?

The response of a concerned individual will help us understand. *"I don't like to see people take chances like that,"* she said, *"I've learned that things can happen."* In other words, she was saying that, based on her previous life experiences, she was scared to watch me hold Brittany in the air, balanced on my hand. She was afraid that I might drop Brittany or that in some way my baby might get hurt.

But what about Brittany? Why did she not react the same

way? The conclusion we must make is that she had no reason to fear. She had an inborn "default setting" that she was safe. There was no reason for her to have an unsafe feeling.

Brittany was born into this world with no fear. A person could hang her from a twenty story building and it wouldn't matter to her. She would feel that she was safe because that is how newborns come into this world. Our older children were quite impressed by the fact that they could wave their hands in front of her face and she wouldn't even blink her eyes. She simply had no fearful response.

THE SAFE AND THE UNSAFE BOX

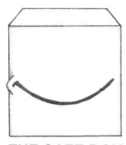 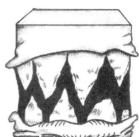

THE SAFE BOX   **THE UNSAFE BOX**

We might say that we each are born into this world with two empty boxes inside our mind. One box is a **Safe Box**; the other is an **Unsafe Box**. Each experience we have in life goes into one of these two boxes. Based on what is in our boxes, we know how to respond to the next similar experience that comes our way. From our story above, we see that Brittany was responding to the experience by feeling safe. That was her default box. She had nothing stored in her Unsafe Box that said standing on Dad's hand was unsafe or dangerous. Therefore, standing on Dad's hand was a safe experience, and perceived as such, allowed her to feel safe when doing it again.

The women, on the other hand, had *"... learned that things can happen."* Based on experiences stored in their Unsafe Boxes, they saw Brittany standing on her Dad's hand as unsafe and dangerous. Why the different reactions?

All of us come into the world the same way as Brittany -

we are all born with a pattern or program in our brain that says we are safe. It is not something we choose, or decide upon. We just are that way. It is innate and natural to us. It is our default setting. However it doesn't take long for that setting to begin to be replaced. Replaced with what?

FEAR BRINGS A TEAR

Let's allow Brittany to teach us again. I noticed one day that Brittany had crawled up onto a big round foam cushion in the middle of our living room floor. It wasn't the first time she had been on the cushion, but this time she reacted differently. The foam was six inches high and she had previously rolled off it several times. This time, after playing for a while on top, she began to cry. She had crawled to the edge but wouldn't go any further. It was obvious to her that she was afraid she was going to fall again.

We see that Brittany now had experience and knowledge on her side. After falling off the edge of the cushion a few times, she recognized the edge as an uncomfortable place to be. She knew it was where a hurtful and startling experience had repeated itself several times, and she had stored that memory in her Unsafe Box. With this new recognition, she did not know how to handle the edge of the cushion, and being afraid of getting hurt again, she cried. I picked her up, gave her a kiss and hug, and she was once again safe and comfortable in her environment.

Fear is the first real negative emotion we feel. As a baby, it may be fear of falling, fear of being left alone, fear of going hungry, fear of rejection, or fear of being injured. Whatever the fear is that we develop, it is based on an experience or experiences that hurt us physically or emotionally, or make us feel unsafe. So we store them in our Unsafe Box. Those experiences teach us that the default setting of safety we are born with doesn't fit the picture anymore. We learn that there are things that hurt, physically and emotionally. Fear is a warning signal to avoid those things so we don't get hurt again.

The women in the class had a reason to fear for Brittany. In their Unsafe Boxes, they had many experiences that said what I was doing to Brittany was unsafe, and there was potential for harm. Brittany didn't have any such experience in her Unsafe Box, so she had no reason to fear. She could stand tall and happy in my hand, and be fearless. Falling off the six inch cushion a couple of times was a different experience, and produced a different kind of reaction. Hurt was introduced, and she had now stored an experience in her Unsafe Box that caused her to be wary of six inch cushions.

TO STAY ALIVE IS OUR STRONGEST DRIVE

The strongest natural instinct humans have is self-preservation. Anything that hurts us is a threat to our very existence. In an effort to avoid that threat, we have a response we call fear. When the possibility of a harmful experience recurs, we feel fear, which causes us to do whatever is necessary to avoid going through the experience a second time. Brittany learned that falling hurts and her survival instinct told her that falling is not a good thing to do again. Therefore, when she approached the edge of the cushion, fear warned her of what could happen, so she started to cry.

Emotional hurts are just as threatening as physical injuries, though maybe not so obvious. They, too, produce fear in a person, which he or she subconsciously makes every effort to avoid.

Grace was divorced after twenty years of marriage, and lost everything important to her in the settlement. She had a good job in a hospital but was not enjoying it. One day she hurt her back lifting a suitcase. It wasn't long before she quit work, giving back pain as her reason. She went and lived with her mother for two years. During that time she very seldom went out of the house. She became very fearful. She would panic if she got very far from home or was out for any length of time. One day she realized how paranoid she had become and decided to force herself to go back to work. She obtained an excellent job but quit after only a couple months. She wasn't sure why.

I explained to Grace how fear could be involved. At one point in her life, before the divorce, she had everything and then lost it. That memory was stored in her Unsafe Box. I suggested that she was possibly afraid to obtain anything again for fear that it would once more be taken away. Therefore, there was no point in working and, as a result, she didn't enjoy her work. Grace felt that this was, indeed, the answer to her paranoia and pain and resolved to change her attitude. She was successfully able to move this experience into her Safe Box and eventually take on and keep another job and be free of pain in her back.

IMAGINATION - A <u>REAL</u> SENSATION

In addition to our Unsafe Box being filled with real physical and emotional threats to our survival, there are also imaginary ones.

Susan was twenty-eight years old and had nightmares three or four times a week. This had been going on for as long as she could remember. When I met her she said that she would often wake up screaming and beating her husband. Those nightmares, while she was having them, were very real to her. The monsters, murderers, and other villains were not real, though she physically reacted as though they actually existed. In fact, the main person experiencing reality was her husband who was getting beaten.

I told Susan that fear was part of her survival mechanism and that some fearful memory from the past was probably responsible for her nightmares now. She told me that she used to watch a lot of horror movies. She also said she was raised on a farm where they had rattlesnakes, and it wasn't uncommon to find one in the house. As a child she would often dream that there was a snake in her bed.

Once Susan understood how her nightmares could be due to her fears, she resolved to work on letting go of their cause and placing them in her Safe Box. She was able to do so and has only had a couple of nightmares since.

§ **How did she do that?**
§ **What's the connection between the mind and the body?**
§ **How is our health affected by our feelings?**
§ **How does fear affect us physically?**

To really understand these questions and others, we need to go back to the beginning – the beginning of us.

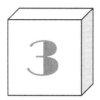

THE BODY AUTOMATIC

THE AUTOMATIC MIRACLE

A human being is the greatest creation on earth. From the moment of conception, the body grows, develops, and functions without the need for conscious thought. What a miracle it is! Respiration, circulation, digestion, assimilation, and other processes run automatically, usually without awareness. For example, the liver performs about five hundred functions that we know of, none of which are under our conscious control. Just being able to stand is an extremely complicated interaction of nerves and muscles. We do all these things with hardly a thought; yet so do all other animals. What makes us different from them? Is it not our capacity to think, reason, and feel? Though some animals may have a minimal capacity to do these same things, our ability is immense.

Suppose a hunter is out chasing a deer. If they both run for two miles their physical reactions would be similar. Their heart rates quicken, their blood pressures increase, and their breathing becomes faster and deeper. When they stop running, their bodily functions return to their normal resting levels.

Compare that to eighty-three year old Mrs. Meyers. She complained that her heart was beating extremely fast, so fast that it frightened her, and it was worse around two o'clock in the morning.

I explained to Mrs. Meyers how the mind can sometimes send a message to the body so it does the right thing at an undesirable time. A fast heart beat is a right and normal thing when the hunter is chasing a deer, but not if he is just sitting. I suggested that stress, and in particular, fear, can be responsible for the undesirable communication between mind and body.

Mrs. Meyers said she knew exactly when the rapid heart beat began. She was having new shingles put on her house and one of the roofers was drunk. His language was very offensive to her and she was afraid that he would do a shoddy job. She was rehearsing in her mind all the reasons why she didn't have to put up with such abuse and how to tell him he was fired.

Can you see why Mrs. Meyers was experiencing fear? She felt that she needed to tell this man to leave, and that was scary for her. She must have had an experience, or experiences, in her Unsafe Box that made her nervous to confront him. Just as Brittany didn't know what to do when she got to the edge of the cushion, Mrs. Meyers was afraid of her next step. If she told him to leave, would he cooperate? Would he use more foul language? Would he hurt her?

Brittany solved her problem by crying. In response to her tears, I picked her up and everything was back to normal. Mrs. Meyer's solution was not that simple. Instead of quickly resolving the problem, she continued to dwell on it. Her fear and the uncertainty of the roofer's response kept her from acting. Instead she dwelt on those feelings and didn't resolve them. She became more and more angry and confused. As a result, her heart started to race.

Why was it that it was her heart that was affected? To understand, we need to better understand the workings of the body.

AUTO PILOT

As indicated earlier, most bodily processes are automatic. Since survival is our strongest instinct, these processes are geared to keep us alive under any circumstance, if at all possible.

There are two important parts to our "survival system". The first involves eating, sleeping, and healing. These are under the control of what is known as the *parasympathetic nervous system*. We could say that this part of survival is working the best when we are at rest or relaxed.

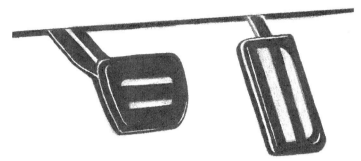

A simple analogy would be to the **brakes** on your car. Pressing the brake pedal is like activating the parasympathetic nervous system. When the parasympathetic nervous system is activated digestion is good, a person sleeps well and healing and repair is normal.

The second part of our "survival system" has to do with activity and emergencies. Our normal daily activities, plus our reaction to anything that threatens us, are mostly controlled by the *sympathetic nervous system*. This would be analogous to the **accelerator** pedal on your car. Pushing on the accelerator would speed up those body processes necessary to run or fight.

There must be a balance between these two parts of the autonomic nervous system (we'll call it the *automatic* nervous system) for the body to work normally. This is done automatically with very little thought or awareness on our part. It is like being on Auto Pilot. If that balance exists, then health also exists as all body processes are generally working as they should.

What I have just described works for humans as well as animals. The deer in the forest is healthy for the same reasons. However, as mentioned earlier, humans have more extensive abilities to think, reason, and feel than animals. We have a mind that permits us, to a certain degree, to override what the body would normally do.

For example, a person can willfully interrupt his normal

pattern of breathing and hold his breath. An animal cannot. Some people can hold their breath for a long time. In fact my nephew can hold his breath until he passes out; however, he cannot hold it until he dies. The body's survival extinct is too strong for that. As soon as he passes out, normal breathing returns.

Let's look, now, at how each of these two systems generally affects the body.

THE ACCELERATOR

Pressing the "accelerator" of the sympathetic nervous system will:

1. Increase blood pressure
2. Increase heart rate
3. Increase circulation
4. Increase muscle tone
5. Increase respiration
6. Increase body metabolism
7. Increase mental activity
8. *Decrease the ability to heal*
9. *Decrease digestion*
10. *Decrease ability to sleep*

THE BRAKE

Pressing the "brake" of the parasympathetic nervous system will do just the opposite.

1. *Decrease blood pressure*
2. *Decrease heart rate*
3. *Decrease circulation*
4. *Decrease muscle tone*
5. *Decrease respiration*
6. *Decrease body metabolism*
7. *Decrease mental activity*
8. Increase the ability to heal
9. Increase digestion
10. Increase ability to sleep

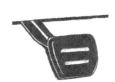

FIGHT OR FLIGHT

To make this a little easier to understand, we might think of the entire concept as a Fight or Flight mechanism.

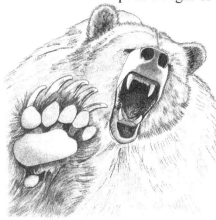

Suppose a bear walked into the room where you are now reading. Imagine what your reactions would be as you hit the "accelerator" to deal with this emergency. By looking at the list, you can easily see why the first seven items would increase and the last three decrease. It wouldn't make much sense to have your digestive processes increasing when you're being attacked.

Your body would go into emergency survival and the sympathetic system would dominate. Once you escape from the bear, flee the house, and find a safe place again, it's easy to see the need for the parasympathetic to take over. You put on the "brake" so the body can slow down, rest and recover. Your Auto Pilot shifts gears. It is necessary to recharge your body for the next activity or emergency. Therefore, we could say that anything that causes a Fight or Flight reaction will trigger a sympathetic nervous system response.

We must remember now, that this is all done automatically. No thinking is involved. A different reaction would occur if you had a pet bear and realized it was only him walking into the room. Your thought would be, *"Oh, it's only my pet bear, Teddy"*. Then your mind would send a signal to the nervous system that everything was okay and **this** bear was not a real threat, since this one was in your Safe Box. You would continue to sit and read in your easy chair with hardly a glitch in your heart beat. Your mind would override your natural reaction. Isn't that fantastic? We are truly amazing creations!

The bear provides us an example of reality. What about its opposite, something imagined?

Let's go back to Susan, the woman who was having nightmares. Her case is opposite to the scenario mentioned above. Just as the pet bear, Teddy, was not a threat to you because of your mind, the imagined "bears" in Susan's dreams, were threats to her, also because of her mind. You are able to sit and read a book when Teddy walks in because you perceive no threat. Susan couldn't even sleep since imminent danger threatened as soon as she closed her eyes. It soon becomes obvious that what we **perceive** as a threat is what our body responds to, whether it is actually a literal threat or not!

Now let's see if we can answer the question we posed earlier, *"Why did Mrs. Meyers' heart begin to beat so fast?"* Maybe it would help if we asked another question first. *"Did Mrs. Meyers perceive a threat?"* Undoubtedly, she did. She was afraid of what the roofer's reaction would be when she asked him to leave. That fear stimulated the sympathetic nervous system just like it is supposed to, and her body responded appropriately with an increased heart rate. The threat was very real to her and she physically reacted to it. How wonderful! Wonderful, because her body was doing exactly what it was told.

Let's discuss another elderly person. *Mr. Moses was eighty-two years old. For three weeks he had been complaining of dizziness. Everything seemed to spin so badly that he frequently needed to lie down. His doctor had prescribed blood pressure medication hoping that it might help, though his blood pressure was relatively normal. Other tests had ruled out tumors. I asked Mr. Moses what he thought the cause of his dizziness was. He said that it was due to stress. He was sure of it. I asked what had happened three weeks earlier that could have brought it on. He was a rancher running thousands of head of sheep and several hundred head of cattle. Much of the land his livestock grazed on was owned by the government. He said that he had a run in with the guys from the Bureau of Land Management (BLM) over some paper work. They had made him angry.*

Did Mr. Moses perceive himself as being threatened? Sure he did. Whether he was actually being threatened or not made little difference. He felt threatened, which hit the accelerator and stimulated the sympathetic nervous system, which automatically produced a physical response.

We mentioned in our bear story that once you escaped the bear and found a safe place again, your parasympathetic nervous system would take over and your body would slow down and rest. You would be ready to digest food, to sleep, or to heal. Now suppose that Mr. Moses continued to think about those "bad" BLM guys that made him angry. Suppose he continued to perceive that he was being threatened by them. Would those thoughts continue to affect him physically? By all means! His body would still do what it had been programmed to automatically do. If his mind was continually sending a signal that he was being threatened, his body would physically react to preserve itself.

Can you see how this temporary emergency reaction could lead to a constant physical manifestation we call a symptom? Can you see why Mrs. Meyers would go to the doctor with a fast heart rate and Mr. Moses would feel dizzy for three weeks?

THE KEY THAT OPENS THE DOOR

Here is the key to many of the health problems we have:

We are reacting to something in our Unsafe Box!

We are reacting to something that we perceive or once perceived as a threat. Again, I must emphasize that it doesn't matter if it was a real threat or not. It's our perception of the situation that is important, and that determines which "Box" the experience is stored in. It also doesn't matter if the situation occurred twenty minutes ago, twenty years ago, or if we think it will happen in the future. Our minds are like a computer in that it doesn't matter when data is entered. Once there, it is stored and ready for recall. We react accordingly until the data is updated, and then we can respond to the updated version. As long as you're afraid there is a bear in the room, your mind will send that message to your body, and your body will automatically produce the appropriate protective response. If you update that information to say that the bear has left, your body will automatically respond differently, whether or not the bear was real or whether or not he actually left.

Hanging on to a perceived threat can lead to any health problem we can imagine. It is responsible for many more of our health concerns and diseases than we are aware. By understanding this fact, we are able to open the door to better health. The two parts of the automatic nervous system we have talked about, the parasympathetic and sympathetic (the brake and the accelerator) run on Auto Pilot according to a perceived need. They must be balanced to be healthy. Our thoughts and fears can interfere with that delicate balance and affect us physically. Symptoms can appear in any part of the body, since the entire body is controlled by the automatic nervous system. Therefore, a person may develop headaches, backaches, depression, anxiety attacks, hormone imbalances, joint pain, gastritis, high blood pressure, diabetes, or tumors; the list is endless.

SURVIVAL REACTIONS

Sarah had been living with debilitating pain in her neck, back, shoulders, and arms for twelve years. She had a difficult time sleeping, and had problems with digestion. The diagnosis she was given was fibromyalgia.

As we apply what we have learned, we might conclude that Sarah's body's physical reactions are coming from some previous experience stored in her Unsafe Box. She started having these symptoms twelve years ago, so the obvious question to ask her was what was going on twelve years earlier in her life.

Sarah knew the answer to that. Her twin sister had died. For most people, that would obviously be a very stressful experience. Natural survival instincts would kick in and muscles would tighten up, sleeping would become difficult, and there would likely be no desire to eat. Sarah was no different than the average person, and had such reactions at the time of her sister's death. However, twelve years had now passed, and she was still in that survival mode. She was still tensed up, still couldn't sleep, and still had digestive problems when she ate.

Sarah was not consciously choosing her debilitating and frustrating symptoms. They were necessary because of how she perceived the loss of her sister. She was completely unaware of the connection between how she felt in the present, and what had happened in the past, and she didn't realize that she could do anything about it. She experienced a great sense of relief just knowing that there was a cause, and a solution. When I saw her a month later, she had hardly any pain, her digestion was significantly better and her ability to sleep was back to where it was before her sister died.

Over thirty years of clinical practice has taught me that virtually ALL chronic health problems have an emotional component associated with them. There is frequently a secondary nutritional component as well, which we will discuss later.

I must reiterate that the body never makes a mistake. It was created perfectly. The body does whatever it does for a reason. It is perfect in its expression of the message it is receiving. If we don't like what our bodies are doing, then we must focus on changing the **cause** of the symptoms. Focusing only on the symptoms is not nearly as effective in the long run as focusing on the cause of those symptoms.

Sarah's physical symptoms are a good example of the body's reaction to stress that triggers a long time survival response. We might say she has been stuck in the same emergency pattern for twelve years. It is impossible to maintain a survival reaction that long without having symptoms like muscle and joint pain.

This little experiment can show you why that is so. Hold one arm straight out to the side of you. Assuming no shoulder problem, that is easy to do. Keep holding it there for a minute. Are you feeling any discomfort yet? Now hold it for another minute. Keep holding it for five minutes. Can you do it? How 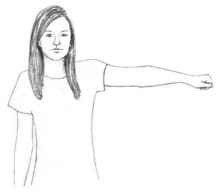 about for ten minutes? For thirty? What about an hour, a week, or a month? How about for twelve years? How long can you hold it out before you are screaming in pain? The shoulder or arm pain you feel is not because there is something wrong with your shoulder or arm. It is simply because the muscles are too tight for too long. When you put your arm down, you get immediate relief.

Can you see how Sarah's muscles had been too tight for

too long? This whole explanation made a lot of sense to Sarah and she was able to face her emotions better and begin healing. She "put her arm down," emotionally speaking, and quickly experienced relief.

Whether it is a death in the family, a dog growling, speaking in public, a car accident, or a myriad of other experiences, survival responses are the same. They are meant to get us away from the threat so we can be safe. Let's look a little closer at a few more of our body's survival reactions, and what may eventually happen if we hang on to them too long.

The chart on the following page shows how the various systems of the body respond to perceived threats.

The Column labeled #1 shows the body's immediate physical reaction to stress, as if a bear suddenly came into the room.

Column #2 shows the symptoms that may develop if the stress is not resolved and the physical reactions continue. It is as if there is always a bear prowling around somewhere, and we never feel safe.

Column #3 lists chronic conditions that could eventually develop as a result of long-term unsafe feelings in Column #2.

BODY'S REACTIONS TRIGGERED BY A FIGHT OR FLIGHT SURVIVAL RESPONSE			
SYSTEM OF THE BODY	1. THE IMMEDIATE REACTION	2. THE LONG TERM REACTION	3. EVENTUAL POSSIBLE CHRONIC CONDITIONS
SKELETAL	Muscles, joints are tense and tight	Muscle pain, spasms, weakness. Joint pain and inflammation.	Fibromyalgia, cramps, tendonitis, arthritis, bursitis, MS, Parkinsons
CIRCULATION	Increased heart rate (need more blood)	Palpitations, arrhythmias	Anxiety, panic attacks, heart failure
	Elevated triglycerides & cholesterol (for energy production)	High triglycerides & cholesterol	Heart disease
	Increased blood pressure (to get more blood to the body)	High blood pressure	Heart disease, stroke
RESPIRATION	Increased (to get more oxygen to body)	Shallow, rapid breathing	Dizziness, asthma
DIGESTION	Slows down (need to run or fight, not digest)	Poor digestion, deficiency of acid and enzymes	Acid reflux, constipation, hiatal hernia
	Speeds up (need to evacuate bowels so can fight)	Rapid digestion, excess acid, frequent bowel movements	Ulcers, diarrhea, IBS, Crohn's
HEALING	Slows down (need to run or fight, not heal)	Weak immune system, injuries slow to heal	Colds, flu, cancer, autoimmune diseases
HORMONES	Increased energy from thyroid & adrenals	Exhaustion as can't run or fight forever	Chronic fatigue, thyroid, adrenal failure
	Decreased reproductive (can't get pregnant when running)	Hormonal imbalances, menstrual irregularities	Decreased sex drive, PMS, sterile, endometriosis
	Increased blood sugar (for energy)	Elevated blood sugar levels	Diabetes
SLEEPING	No desire for sleep (need to fight)	Inability to go to sleep or stay asleep, though tired	Exhaustion, fatigue
	Sleep all the time (need to escape)	Never can get enough sleep	Exhaustion, fatigue
MENTAL	Increased mental acuity (need to solve problem)	Think too much, mind races, can't turn mind off	Anxiety, panic attacks, ADHD, bipolar
	Decreased mental acuity (need to escape)	Depression, discouragement as no solution	Depression, bipolar, suicidal

FEARFUL CONSEQUENCES

If we analyze the thoughts and feelings that are the cause of the body reactions we don't like, we find that they are all negative. Fear, anger, jealousy, revenge, greed, guilt, hate, worry, rejection, selfishness, judgment, and many others will eventually unbalance the nervous system. Of these feelings, fear is primary; all the others are secondary. It is the fear of what people think, the fear of failure, the fear of missing out, the fear of physical or emotional pain, etc. that is the problem.

However, fear is not necessarily always bad. It can be used in a positive way provided it is temporary and we use it to handle the situation. Jumping out of the way of an oncoming car, avoiding a dark alley, or even paying taxes on time can be motivated by fear. But when we continue to hang on to the fear, it will eventually tilt our automatic nervous system out of balance, and a normal body reaction becomes an unwanted symptom.

Jeff was the star of his high school basketball team, averaging twenty points a game. His back was hurting so he came to my office for help. Jeff didn't remember doing anything specifically to hurt it. It just started hurting.

As we talked, it became apparent that Jeff's back was tense due to fear. He was afraid he wasn't doing well enough, that he wasn't meeting the expectations of others and especially himself. There was a lot of pressure on him to perform well. His back muscles had been too tense for too long and he had started to hurt. Figuratively, as described in our experiment earlier, "he needed to put his arm down". Once Jeff understood why his body was doing what it was, he was able to lighten up and not dwell on the pressure or expectations. He finished out the season without any more back problems.

Stress like Jeff felt can have a powerful effect on us. Suppose that you are in charge of the laundry in your house. You are behind schedule and the kids have no clothes to wear to school tomorrow. You put a load of wash in after supper and turn on the machine. You hear a clank and the washer stops. It won't start again. What is your reaction?

This is how Norma reacted. Her first thought was, *"Great! Now what? We don't have any money for a new washing machine!"* Suddenly the memories began to come back to her. She remembered when she lived in a tiny little town in a tiny little house with no running water and no money. She especially recalled having to wash diapers by hand. *"There's no way I'm going through that again,"* she thought. *"That was a horrible experience."* The next morning she awoke with a terrible cough, the same terrible cough she used to have when she lived in that tiny little house. She also had the same terrible heartburn, only worse than before.

Your reaction would probably not have been nearly as severe as Norma's. The idea of being without a washing machine was very frightening to her, due to her previous experience.

You will also notice how quickly Norma developed symptoms. These were not due to the stress of the washing machine breaking down – there had not been enough time for that. The symptoms were due to a **pattern** that had previously been established by a past experience stored in her Unsafe Box.

PERFECT PATTERNS

One of the miracles of the body automatic is its ability to establish patterns. What we persist in doing becomes easier and easier to do, or, as we often hear, practice makes perfect. The more we do something, the more engrained it becomes in both the mind and the physical body. This not only applies to things like learning to play the piano, but also in how we handle stress. Once we have found a way to relieve fear, we will use it again the next time fear comes along. If it works well again, the pattern becomes more established and will be even easier to use a third time. Norma's symptoms appeared as quickly as they did because they were part of a pattern for handling fear that she had established a long time earlier. Though the symptoms were brought on through a subconscious process, the physical reactions were very real.

Lilly's story makes this process even more clear.

Lilly was the mother of ten children and had experienced fourteen pregnancies. Every time she got pregnant, she would develop sciatic pain in her leg during the first month of pregnancy. By the fifth month, the pain would go away. This leg pain did not occur with just one or two pregnancies, but with each of the fourteen pregnancies!

It was obvious that sciatic leg pain during pregnancy was normal for Lilly. But such a pain should never be normal, unless something had caused that pattern to become necessary.

I asked Lilly about her first pregnancy. She'd had the leg pain as mentioned, and the pregnancy ended in a miscarriage. I asked how she felt about that event at the time and she said it was very difficult for her. She said that her younger sister already had two children, and it felt so unfair to her that her sister should be "ahead" of her. She felt like a failure for having a miscarriage, and that she was a disappointment to her husband who was also anxiously looking forward to having a baby. Can you see what was happening here?

So I asked about her second pregnancy. Again she experienced the sciatica in her leg, not surprising considering her previous experience, but not necessarily a pattern at this point. How this pregnancy turned out would likely have a great influence on the pattern for future pregnancies. Lilly said this second pregnancy ended in a still born birth at five months, a much more difficult experience than the first. Lilly's fears of failure and loss had been confirmed, and the pattern was now set and every subsequent pregnancy began with sciatic leg pain. Interestingly, the pain disappeared in the fifth month of pregnancy. Any guesses as to why? It's likely that at that point Lilly was able to let go of her fears of not being able to carry the baby to term. Had Lilly's second pregnancy ended with a healthy baby, it is likely she would not have developed the sciatica in pregnancy pattern.

Chad had symptoms much worse than Norma's or Lilly's. He had severe chest pains off and on over many years. Four or five times they had been bad enough to put him in the hospital in intensive care. Many tests and specialists had failed to find a definitive cause for his pain.

After Chad's most recent attack, he and I determined that he was following a pattern. It appeared that each time he experienced an episode of chest pain, he had been under stress. He would be very busy, to the point of being overwhelmed with what he had to do. Fear that he could not get it all done would set in. Ironically, a solution that would relieve the fear was to have chest pain. Why? Other people would not expect Chad to do all those things he was committed to do when they learned he was having heart problems.

Now, it's important to note, Chad was not doing this consciously. He did not think, *"I believe I will have a heart attack so that I don't have to do all these things."* It was just a pattern that his mind and body had developed to deal with stress. It had become a normal pattern for him. Why this pattern appeared is the subject of the next chapter.

Now let's summarize what we have learned about the body automatic.

1. **Self-preservation is our most driving instinct.**
2. **Most of our body's functions are automatic.**
3. **Our thoughts can override what the body would normally do.**
4. **The parasympathetic and sympathetic nervous systems run on Auto Pilot and must be balanced for normal health.**
5. **Hanging on to perceived threats in our Unsafe Box imbalances our automatic nervous system and leads to symptoms.**
6. **Fear is the major perceived threat.**
7. **The mind and body develop patterns to deal with stress.**

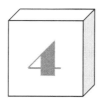

WHAT YOU THINK
IS WHAT YOU GET

"What you see is what you get" is a cute little phrase that is familiar to most of us. A more profound one might be *"What you **think** is what you get."* Positive thinkers have told us that for years. Whether the thought is positive or negative, thinking it is a good way to bring it about.

We concluded the previous chapter by talking about Chad. His chest pain was a pattern his mind and body had developed when he was feeling overwhelmed. Some experience in the past had caused his automatic nervous system to become unbalanced. A perceived threat, now stored as a memory in his Unsafe Box, had stimulated his sympathetic nervous system, creating an expected increased contraction of the heart muscle. That was a normal, natural and necessary reaction. However, Chad continued to hang on to this "threat", and the normal and necessary reaction eventually produced a symptom of severe chest pain. That reaction then became a pattern Chad developed when feeling over-stressed.

THE GREAT (EMOTIONAL) ESCAPE

If you had a task to do, and could not do it, which option would you prefer as the reason for failing?

1. You were not physically capable.
2. You were not emotionally capable.

Most people would choose option 1, not physically capable. It is easier to explain and better understood than not emotionally capable. Not only do we choose that consciously, but it seems we choose that subconsciously as well. Chad subconsciously chose "not physically capable" when his overwhelming emotional load manifested itself as chest pain. Chest pain is an acceptable reason for failing. Emotional overload, or too much to do, is not.

There are two points that need to be emphasized here.

1. Emotional or mental stress is often more difficult to bear than physical pain.

Thus, emotional stress is often "transferred" or "escapes" to the physical body, even though that may mean a physical symptom. That symptom can be anything in any part of us. It may be anything from acne to yeast infections and everything in between. Chad's chest pain was actually easier for him to deal with than an emotional load that wouldn't go away. He was able to go to the hospital to obtain physical relief. There was no where to go for emotional relief. It just continued to increase.

2. Other people can relate to a physical problem better than an emotional one, making a physical ailment more "acceptable".

Emotionally Chad felt "safer" with chest pain as his problem, than saying his problem was that he couldn't do everything. He had a tangible explanation he could give to people. Again, this happened without conscious thought. It was automatic. So Chad's emotional stress "escaped" to his body, where he could justify to himself and to others his reason for not getting it all done.

Barbara's story reinforces this concept that emotional stress escapes to the physical body.

Barbara was a book publisher and had a publishing deadline and a child getting married one week apart. The stress to get an extremely long list of things done was overwhelming and she ended up in bed for five days with terrible back pain.

Can you see why?

Considering the points above, the emotional stress of being overwhelmed with too much to do escaped to, or was transferred to her back. The emotional stress was literally easier for her to handle there. She could thus justify to herself, and to her boss and son why she was not able to get everything done. That was a reason with which she could live.

Remember, this happens automatically, without conscious thought. It is how our mind and body work together. The physical pain is "safer" than the emotional burden. So the great emotional escape is to the physical body. This is extremely common and it happens to everyone.

Walter was sixty-five years old. He came into my office using two canes, walking on his tiptoes. The back of his legs were drawn up so tightly his heels would not touch the floor. He had been like this for seven years, and had not been able to work. Walter said that seven years earlier he had back surgery. His back did really well after the surgery. Then, two months later when it was time to go back to work, the backs of his legs drew up, and he never did return to work. He had been on disability since.

I asked Walter why he had back surgery in the first place. His bottom-line answer was revealing. He actually said, *"I despised my boss, and did it to get out of work."* I knew then that there was nothing I could do to "fix" him. He was going to have to fix himself. When I explained to Walter what he would need to do, he wasn't interested. His emotional duress with his boss had lead to back pain, and ultimately his disability. But he was not willing to forgive or let go and move on. So there was nothing I could do to help him.

Now let me emphasize that transferring emotional stress to the physical body is not bad. It's normal; it's according to our natures and each one of us does it. Like water flowing downhill, it naturally goes this way and is difficult to stop. However, this transfer is not necessary! There is a better way. It takes effort, but the rewards are worth it.

NO FOOLIN'!

What we think is what we get. Can you see how Barbara was thinking, *"There's too much to do! I've got too big a load to carry! I'm overwhelmed! I'll never get it all done!"*

Can you see why it affected her back? The ever increasing fear of failing to be ready for the wedding and the publishing deadline unbalanced the automatic nervous system. The thought of not being able to carry it all dictated which part of that system would be most affected. It's logical that it would be her back since she had too much "weight on her back". Like our experiment of holding your arm out too long, it is just a matter of time before the emergency response could become a symptom. It's also easy to see how lifting a five pound weight or even bending over to tie a shoe could then be "the straw that broke the camel's back".

As we resolve our stresses, we need to understand what our thoughts and feelings are about those stresses. There is more we can learn from Chad's experience. When did he first start having chest pains, and what stressful situation was going on at the time?

Chad says that the chest pains began when he was married to his first wife. Things weren't going very well between them when he had his first episode. He remembered thinking, *"If I die, then she'll **really** feel bad!"* Again we can see that the prolonged stress, as would occur in a difficult relationship, would eventually unbalance the automatic nervous system. The thought of dying, or even the effect of having an emotionally broken heart over his relationship, could very easily direct the physical heart to be the area most affected. Thus a pattern was begun.

Though thinking about dying as a cause of chest pain may seem a little drastic, it can and does work that way. It is impossible to lie to or joke with ourselves. Everything we sincerely think or feel is accepted and recorded as the truth.

When we understand this fact, we can then see how destructive our thoughts can really be. *"I'm ugly"*, *"I can't do anything right"*, *"I'm scared to death"*, *"Mondays are the worst day of the week"*, *"I can't stand it"*, *"That gives me a headache"*, *"That's hard to swallow"*, *"I'm falling apart"*, *"It comes with old age"*, etc., are not harmless phrases. Our body accepts them as facts from our mind and goes to work to make them a reality. The body is just doing what it is being told.

It's not just our thoughts that can be destructive; our words often are too. Though obviously there has to be some thought before word patterns begin, we often fall into the trap of using expressions that have a negative impact on us, like the ones listed above. We can easily get into a destructive habit of saying negative things about ourselves or the situation we are in.

I had a simple experience years ago that taught me this lesson. Three of my children and I were having fun at the kitchen counter making pita bread. At least it was fun until the teasing and poking and prodding began. I finally became exasperated with my five year old who wouldn't stop his antics. I said, *"Stop that! I am really <u>tired</u> of you doing that! I mean it! Stop it right now!"*

Can you see what I had done to myself? I had said that I was really tired! I didn't just leave it at that, but reinforced it by saying, *"I mean it!"* Do you think those words could affect me physically, especially if my son ignored me and continued to do it anyway? In five minutes I actually felt a deep sense of heaviness behind my eyes and thought that I could use a nap. I thought it was kind of odd how quickly that sleepiness had come on in the middle of a project. It was then I realized what I had done to myself physically by what I had thought and said.

WHAT COMES FROM ME BECOMES ME

Write down or make a mental list of five expressions you often use. They may be like those listed above – *"I can't stand it"*, *"That makes me sick"*, *"It's a real pain"*, etc. Think about how the expression would affect you physically if taken literally.

Expressions Used

1._____

2._____

3._____

4._____

5._____

Trish was a nineteen year old university student who had just completed her second semester. She came in to see me saying that she was sick all the time. The past four months she had continuously been on antibiotics. Not only that, but she could sleep sixteen hours and still wake up tired. I asked her if she enjoyed school. She said no; that she was sick and tired of it. I asked her if there was anything else she was "sick and tired" of. There was. She was sick and tired of not having enough money. In fact, she was quitting school and was going to be a nanny.

I explained to Trish the mind-body connection. She found this enlightening and could readily see what she was doing to herself. She made the necessary mental changes and within a few days was feeling like her normal self again. Interestingly she later became a fire jumper, something much more suited to her personality and talents.

DOUBLE MINDED IN ALL OUR WAYS

The body acts upon the information it receives from the mind. Let me explain further.

There are two main parts to the mind, the *subconscious* and the *conscious*. The subconscious is the part we cannot deceive. It accepts everything entered into it as fact, for it does not have the ability to reason. It is responsible for the automatic functioning of the body. We therefore need to be careful what we put into the subconscious since that information will be integrated into the "programming" which runs the body.

The conscious mind is the reasoning part. This is like a filter through which all information must pass before it can enter the subconscious. If accepted by the conscious mind, information moves on and is stored by the subconscious. If rejected by the conscious, then the subconscious doesn't even have the opportunity to see it.

There are two ways information can get through the conscious mind and be stored in the subconscious mind. One is through frequency. The more often a thought occurs, the more readily it is accepted, until it is believed to be true. It doesn't matter whether it is really true or not. We all know people who call black, white and white, black. They may not be obstinate, but may actually have said it or thought it enough to believe it. Therefore an innocent *"I can't stand it"*, said often enough, may lead to a foot, knee, leg, or back problem that doesn't allow the person to stand.

Phil hobbled into my office. He said, *"Doc, you need to x-ray my knee and fix it. I can hardly walk."* *"What did you do?"* I asked. *"Nothin','"* Phil responded, *"I just helped someone move a few things, and then it started hurting'."* Because he had no real physical cause, I asked him if there was something happening in his life that was stressful. *"Yeah,"* he said, *"I **can't stand** the guy my daughter's dating. And my other daughter came home with her kid, and that's a stress. Doc, my family's just falling apart."*

I told Phil that if he had been thinking these thoughts very much lately, they sure could be the reason for his pain. We then talked about what he needed to do to change his way of thinking. He was able to apply some of it right there as we talked, and by the time he left the office, his knee was eighty percent better. It soon healed completely and required no further treatment.

The first way information enters the subconscious mind is through frequency, or repetition of thoughts and words. The second way information enters is through our emotions. The more often we feel something, or the more deeply we feel it, the more easily it enters our subconscious mind. Feelings are not subject to being filtered like our thoughts, but have a direct route into this part of our "computer". As a result they are more powerful than our thoughts.

Erma was a very active sixty-five-year-old woman. A year before coming to see me she had fallen off a stool and hurt her hip and shoulder. The hip healed but the shoulder never did. In fact, it was extremely difficult for her to even raise her arm.

When we consider the automatic ability of her body to heal, we must conclude that something was interfering with that normal process. If everything was working as it should, her shoulder should have healed just as her hip had. In an effort to determine what was interfering, I asked Erma if she remembered what she thought as she fell. She said, *"Probably, 'Oh, you dummy!'"* I explained to her how thoughts can sometimes interfere with the normal healing process. She said, *"Oh, I think that thought all the time. In fact my husband calls me a dummy every day. I can never do anything right for him. I don't know why I bother to stay with the man."*

Let's see if we can apply what we have learned to Erma. We said that both thoughts and feelings send information to the subconscious part of the mind, and that the subconscious is responsible for the automatic functioning of the body. What thought is Erma sending to her subconscious? *"I'm a dummy."* Is she sending it frequently? Yes, several times a day with the help of her husband. She probably really felt dumb when she fell. So something as foolish as falling off a stool reinforced that thought.

Are feelings involved? From the few words she said, we can determine that she must have some very negative feelings about her husband and also about herself. Are her thoughts and feelings interfering with her body's ability to heal? Yes, definitely. How? When Erma thinks of herself as a dummy, she also subconsciously recalls falling off the stool. That reminds her that she has a bad shoulder. If she reminds herself several times a day that she's a dummy, she also keeps recalling the thought that she has a bad shoulder. Therefore it never has a chance to heal. We might say that "dummy" and "bad shoulder" are programmed together on the same track in her brain. The one now automatically goes with the other, and as long as she continues to have the negative thought, she will continue to have the symptom.

Erma was determined to change her thoughts and feelings so that her shoulder could heal. When I saw her five days later, she was much, much better. She said that changing her attitude was making a big difference. She also said that she had made a mistake at work one evening and thought, *"Oh, you dummy!"* Immediately she got a shot of pain in that shoulder, so she was certain that we were treating the correct cause.

A PICTURE, WORTH A THOUSAND WORDS

Many years ago I heard the following analogy. I don't know its source, but it really helped me at the time to understand the difference between the subconscious and conscious minds.

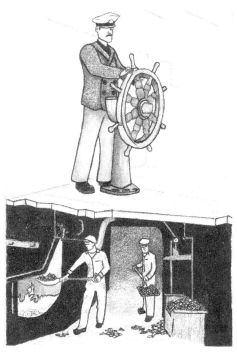

Our conscious mind is like the captain of a steam ship. The captain sees and controls everything. He is in charge. He determines how fast and in what direction the ship is to be going. He sends this information to the members of the crew down below. They are like the subconscious. They take the information from the captain and apply it. If the captain says to go faster, they put more coal in the fire. If he says to slow down, they cut down the steam. Whether his decisions are good or bad, or right or wrong, cannot be determined by the crew. They just do what they are told.

The ship then is like the body. The ship responds to the workings of the members of the crew and carries them in the direction and speed that the captain has chosen.

HOW WE DEAL WITH WHAT WE FEEL

Sometimes we may not be able to describe our sentiments in words, we just feel them.

Kaye's complaint was that, for several months, she'd had a pressure or pain in her low back and down her right leg. At times it was a nagging ache, at other times it was severe. She also had a stiff neck that had bothered her for years. Two months before I saw her she had undergone a hysterectomy.

Kaye was under pressure. She didn't know how else to describe what she was feeling other than that she was just under a lot of pressure. Most of it she thought was due to her husband. A few months earlier he had walked off his job complaining that he didn't like what his employers were doing. That was a fairly consistent pattern for him; it had happened several times before. He was a good, compassionate man, just not very responsible. That left Kaye feeling the pressure of mounting unpaid bills and family responsibilities. She said it seemed as though they were just able to crawl out of one hole long enough to crawl into another one. Her husband was also in trouble with the law. She had thought of divorce, but she loved him. She just wished she could get him to change.

It's easy to see why Kaye felt that she was under pressure, and how that could manifest as pressure in her back. When she went to the doctor, he told her that her uterus was swollen and was putting pressure on the nerves in her low back, and that this was the cause of her back and leg pain. A hysterectomy was performed. Two months later there was still very little improvement in the pain and pressure in her back. I explained to Kaye her feelings could be the cause of her symptoms, and may have contributed to the enlarged uterus originally. The key to her healing was changing her attitude and accepting her husband as he was. Though it was a difficult challenge for her, there weren't any other options that looked any better. She was able to work on that, make that change and totally relieve herself of her chronic symptoms. (Part 2 will explain how she made that change.)

Now let's consider another patient.

Martha was divorced, about thirty-eight years old, and had three children. She was much heavier than she wished to be and wanted some help to lose weight.

Martha and I talked about the weight loss programs she had tried and her lack of success. I explained how the body works automatically and that if she were doing the right things her body would go to its normal and proper weight. We discussed her diet and decided that logically, she wasn't eating enough to be as heavy as she was. I explained to her how thoughts and feelings can interfere with what the body would normally and logically do, which could possibly be giving her a weight problem. She said, *"I've wondered about that. A man called me the other day and asked me out to lunch. I didn't want to go with him and I declined the invitation. As soon as I hung up the phone, I went and ate a peanut butter and jelly sandwich. I don't know why I did. I wasn't even hungry."*

Can you figure out Martha's problem? Why did she eat the sandwich? What might she be thinking or feeling that would cause such a response?

Martha was able to figure it out herself. She said that she was afraid to get into a relationship with another man. She had been through several bad experiences in the past and didn't want to go through them again. If she was overweight, men would not find her attractive and she wouldn't have to worry about a relationship developing. A phone call from a man must, in a sense, have meant it was time to eat again. She was also afraid that she didn't have time for her children as well as a relationship. She feared that if a relationship did develop, she would neglect her children. She didn't want that to happen. This worry, along with the fear of having a relationship with a man affected her subconsciously and she ate to "protect" herself.

CONSCIOUS INPUT

So the subconscious mind has one major function in addition to survival:

1. **Survival.**
2. **Storage of important information.**

Our bodies can then run on auto pilot as much as possible. That way we can tie our shoes or drive a car without having to relearn how each time we make the attempt. We don't have to think about and choose every action, but can react virtually immediately. What a wonderful, efficient system that is!

The marvelous gift of a conscious mind, on the other hand, has two major functions:

1. **Solve and create**
2. **Defend and protect**.

Our thoughts generally fall into the above two categories. To solve and create is typically a positive response and requires effort; to defend and protect is typically negative and comes naturally.

Barry fell down a flight of stairs three months ago and injured his ankle. It hurt for him to walk, and he couldn't turn it at all without pain. It was not improving, and had become worse the past few days.

If something is not healing as quickly as it should, I always ask about the patient's state of mind. The fact that he was still hurting told me that he was still defensive and protective of whatever happened in that fall. He must have put it in his Unsafe Box. Falling down the stairs might indicate that someone else was involved. So I asked him if he had blamed anyone else for what happened.

Barry admitted that he had been pushed. I explained to him how he could not possibly get well until he was able to see that experience differently, let it go, and store it in his Safe Box. He was able to do so. When he got off the table, he was able to stand and turn his foot without any pain. The relief was immediate, as there was nothing to heal. He had to quit defending and protecting himself from something no longer present.

The "defend and protect" component is quick and automatic. The "solve and create" portion usually takes time, effort and thought.

Survival reactions are automatic, yet whether or not they remain is a choice. Remember Sarah, whose twin sister passed away? Sarah had either not been able to, or had chosen not to be at peace with her sister's death. She continued to see it as bad and wrong, something to defend against. Such reconciliation can be a very difficult thing to accomplish. Sarah had to judge it differently if she wanted to be free of the pain she was experiencing. She needed to see that she had a problem she needed to solve, not something to defend against.

When an animal in the wild is threatened, its survival instinct tells it whether to run or fight. When the threat is gone, the animal returns to its normal pattern of living. Animals do not fret about what has happened in the past, or worry about what will happen in the future. They live second to second, moment to moment, always based on what is happening in the present.

Human beings are not that simple. Because of our creative conscious mind we can dwell on the past and live in fear of the future. In fact it is difficult for many of us to simply enjoy the present. It is literally a choice whether we do or not. Sarah is a good example of one who was not living in the present. Unlike the deer that can go back to lazily grazing after it has been chased by a hunter, Sarah's conscious mind kept her in a tense state of survival. Why was it doing this? Why couldn't she just let go?

Richard's story will help. I have known Richard for at least twenty years. He has fought with high blood pressure the entire time I have known him. A few years ago he suffered a heart attack. He will readily tell you why he had high blood pressure and what caused his heart attack. It was his job. He faced deadlines every day and worked with others who faced similar daily deadlines. He constantly felt overwhelmed and threatened. The pressure of meeting his deadlines, and dealing with others trying to meet theirs was always intense. He was certain that this was the cause of his heart problems. One day he decided to quit his job. So he did. He didn't have another job to go to, which also frightened him, but he quit anyway.

How do you think he felt the day he quit his job? Relieved and free, or nervous and fearful? Richard actually felt relieved. He felt safe and free. His blood pressure came down, and other physical symptoms disappeared as well. What about the fact that he didn't have another job? That didn't matter, at least at that moment. He was just happy to be free. Richard was able to use his conscious mind to find a solution to his problem.

His feelings changed, and his body's reactions changed for the better.

Richard had felt unsafe about his job for twenty years, so he had the same survival reaction of high blood pressure for twenty years. When he quit his job, he was free from the threat. He used his conscious mind to judge the experience of <u>not</u> having a job as <u>non</u>-threatening, even though most of us would see being without a job as a greater threat. Because he made that judgment as non-threatening, he felt "safe" and his body reacted accordingly and his blood pressure went down. Twenty years of experience taught him that his job was actually more scary than being unemployed. It took twenty years, but his perspective changed.

Sarah's perspective also needed to change before she could get well. That was not easy. Her conscious mind was keeping her in a tense state of survival. To accept the death of her sister in a positive way was difficult, like quitting a job before you have another. There is something counter-intuitive about that. Sometimes we just have to make the choice that seems to be right and act on that. Sarah was able to do that, and that is the reason her symptoms went away.

We've mostly discussed negative thoughts and feelings so far. This was necessary in order to understand the power of their influence. Negative thoughts and feelings are very often the cause of the health problems we have. What is even more important is to understand their opposites, the power of positive thoughts and feelings. The following chapters will explain these concepts.

Let's summarize what we have learned in this chapter.

1. **What we think and say is what we get.**
2. **The mind will "relieve" stress by transferring it to the body.**
3. **The subconscious accepts all feelings and thoughts that enter it as true, whether they are or not.**
4. **The conscious mind filters and selects information. It solves and creates, defends and protects.**
5. **Our nature is to handle stress negatively. It takes an effort to be positive.**

SUGGESTION: Choose one negative phrase that you frequently use. You might ask someone who knows you well what phrase you say all the time. (Examples: *"I give up"*, *"What if"*, *"It makes me sick"*, *"I can't stand it"*, *"I could just die"*, *"You're a pain in the neck"*, *"I'm afraid"*, *"I'm so tired of it"*). You may want to use one of the five you listed earlier.

Resolve to do away with this phrase and just see what happens!

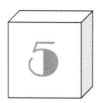

TURN ON THE LIGHTS

IT'S NO BIG DEAL!

The movie, *Home Alone*, contained a scene that teaches a valuable lesson. Kevin, a seven year old, and his neighbor, Old Man Marley, were seated on a church pew. The old man is saying that he is not welcome with his son. Their conversation proceeds like this:

Marley: *Years back, before you and your family moved on the block, I had an argument with my son.*

Kevin: *How old is he?*

Marley: *He's grown up. We lost our tempers. I told him I didn't care to see him anymore. He said the same. We haven't spoken to each other since.*

Kevin: *If you miss him, why don't you call him?*

Marley: *I'm afraid if I call him, he won't talk to me.*

Kevin: *How do you know?*

Marley: *I don't know. I'm just afraid he won't.*

Kevin: *No offense, but, aren't you a little old to be afraid?*

Marley: *You can be a little old for a lot of things. You're never too old to be afraid.*

Kevin: *That's true. I've always been afraid of our basement. It's dark. There's weird stuff down there, and it smells funny. That sort of thing. It's bothered me for many years.*

Marley: *Basement's are like that.*

Kevin: *Then I made myself go down there and do some laundry and I found out it's not so bad. All this time I've been worrying about it, but if you turn on the lights, it's no big deal.*

Marley: *What's your point?*

Kevin: *My point is, you should call your son.*

Marley: *What if he won't talk to me?*

Kevin: *At least you'll know. Then you can stop worrying about it. And you won't have to be afraid anymore.*

In the movie Kevin teaches an important lesson to Marley, one which applies very much to us all. ***"If you turn on the lights, it's no big deal."***

He then explains why. ***"At least you'll know. Then you can stop worrying about it. And you won't have to be afraid anymore."***

Such is the case with every fear, worry, stress, or concern we have. Kevin tells Marley that the fear and worry about how his son will react is a whole lot worse than the finding out. By calling his son, he turns on the lights, and then he can really see what is going on. If his son still rejects him, at least it's a fact and not something he is imagining. If his son accepts him, what a blessing! In both cases he conquers his fear, and it no longer has a strong hold on him.

Every stress we face must be handled the same way, by turning on the lights. When we clearly see what we are facing, we can resolve the problem. When the view of our problem is vague or unclear, it can often appear to be much more frightening than it really is, like the basement. This method applies to handling stress of every kind. It may be problems with children, a spouse, money, business, health, injuries, retirement, or death. Shedding light on the problem is necessary to overcoming it.

Kelly had a pain in her left shoulder for several years. Some days were worse than others, but she really noticed it when she rode in the car. If she went on a drive for more than an hour it would severely ache.

As Kelly and I talked about her problem, I asked her if

she had ever been in an accident before, or if riding in a car scared her. She said that she had been in a couple of minor mishaps but nothing serious. However, icy roads did frighten her, and she didn't like driving downhill, as she felt less in control. On-coming cars were especially frightening. She said that she had skidded off an icy road before, and once a drunk had run her off the road. She then said something enlightening, *"You know,"* she said, *"I never really thought about it before, but every time we leave town, I always wonder to myself if this is it, if we'll never come back. It sounds kind of crazy, but maybe that is my problem."*

The light had been turned on. Kelly now knew what was responsible for at least part of her symptoms. As she knew the cause, she could begin to work on the cure. She had wondered if her shoulder ached because of a tumor. Now frightening thoughts of tumors and other "basement" fears were no longer necessary since she could see and understand what was happening. The solution was in sight. Her shoulder rarely gave her problems after that.

BUMPY RIDES

In this book we are primarily concerned with resolving negative emotional stress and memories to improve health. So far, we have learned how the physical body responds to stress and why symptoms develop. We have seen how negative thoughts and feelings will eventually interfere with the normal automatic body functions and lead to pain and disease. Positive thoughts and feelings will do the opposite. Positive thoughts and feelings will enable the body to work normally, and health will be the natural result. When we turn the light on any stress, we observe that we have two options. We see that we can handle the stress either positively or negatively. We either put it in the Safe Box or the Unsafe Box. Marion Hanks told a story that illustrates this principle.

"A father was on an airplane on a short business trip. He had with him his five year old son. He was almost wishing his son was not there as it was a very rough trip. There were down drafts and up drafts, headwinds alternating with tail winds, and some passengers were feeling a bit queasy. Apprehensively, the

father glanced at his son and found him grinning from ear to ear. 'Dad,' he said, 'do they do this just to make it fun for the kids?'" (Marion D. Hanks, "Changing Channels," *Ensign*, Nov 1990, 38)

Both father and son were having the same experience. The father chose to live it negatively; the son chose to live it positively. Now let's turn the light a little brighter on this experience. As we do so, we are able to answer two important questions, **"What am I afraid of?"** and **"Why am I afraid?"**

We know the father must have reacted the way he did based on thoughts of what could happen. Possibly he had previously had a bad flying experience, or was aware of fatal plane crashes. The son probably had no such former experience to base his reaction on. Now, who was right in his response?

They were both right, were they not? They were both responding based on what they had learned in life, and that's how it should be.

MORNING RATTLESNAKES

Let's look at each of them individually. The son had no reason to fear. Consider the following. Do you check the floor beside your bed each morning to make sure you don't step on a rattlesnake? Probably not. What if you had stepped on one when you got out of bed this morning? Would you check the floor tomorrow? Sure, and for quite some time. The son had not seen any rattlesnakes. In other words, he had no reason to be afraid of flying.

The father, we might say, had stepped on a rattlesnake. His response to a rough plane ride may have been appropriate. But suppose that all plane rides frightened him. Then he would be responding inappropriately as the majority of flights are safe. He would need to turn the light on his fear and begin to choose the positive rather than the negative path. By so doing, he could be relieved of the fear he was carrying, just like Marley in *Home Alone*.

We can see what the father in this story was afraid of and possibly why. Whatever the reason, turning the light on by determining what and why the fear exists, is a major step in overcoming it.

FAITH AND FEAR

When we turn the light on our stress, no matter what it is, we can see that we are handling it positively or negatively. If we look even more closely we can see that **positive and negative actually mean faith and fear.** Faith and fear are opposites. We either choose to act with faith that all is well, or choose to act out of fear. It is our choice. We do make that choice, whether we are aware of it or not.

Every day life presents us with hundreds of opportunities to choose. The one choice we are not given is whether we want to choose or not. Being born gives us the right to choice and the obligation to use it. We might as well choose with faith.

Robert was thirty-five years old and had a responsible position in his community. He came to see me after six months of low back pain, which began after lifting a small stack of papers. Surgery had been suggested as a possible alternative, but he wanted to avoid it if he could. Robert said he had a very stressful job, but he thought he handled it well. The mayor, city council, and county commissioners were all his bosses. Any decision he made was liked by some members of the community and disliked by others. Of course, as seems to be the case with the majority of public offices, what he heard most were the dislikes.

The chiropractic adjustments we gave Robert helped some, but he still occasionally had a nagging pain in his lower back. One day, when it was especially bad and he couldn't even bend over to pet the dog, we talked about faith and fear. I said that lifting a stack of papers never should have hurt his back in the first place, but it could have if he was already carrying a heavy mental load. As Robert thought about it, he realized he was not handling the stress nearly as well as he thought. He was much more negative than he believed and concluded he needed to replace those fear thoughts with faith. Instead of fearing what others might think, he focused on doing the best job he could, and having faith in himself. What others thought of him was not that important, as long as he was doing his best. When he came back in a couple of days later, I asked him if he could pet the dog. He replied that it was no problem. He acknowledged that he had seen the light and that a change in attitude was what he needed.

YELLOW LIGHTS

Recognizing stress as causing part of our health problems is not always an easy thing to do. However, there are a few indicators we can use. We gave a list in Chapter 3 of ten systems in our body and how they react to stress. Three of those are controlled by the parasympathetic nervous system. They will decrease or shut down when responding to stress. If we pay attention to them, they can serve as a warning to us. Just as a yellow light warns us that the traffic light will turn red, these three indicators warn us that stress may be the cause of our symptoms.

1. The Yellow Light of Sleep.

Sleeping time is the best healing time, and we need to sleep well to heal well. If we can't go to sleep easily, if we wake up often, if we wake up more tired than when we went to bed, or if we have to sleep more than eight hours to feel rested, it's likely that we are in the Unsafe Box in a fight or flight survival state. When we lie down at night the parasympathetic nervous system should take over for a good night's rest. If we are handling stress with fear instead of faith, then the sympathetic nervous system will still be dominant, focusing on the perceived threat that we talked about previously, and disrupt our sleep. Who wants to sleep when a bear is attacking? If we run from that imaginary bear day after day, month after month, or year after year, we will ultimately be exhausted no matter how much sleep we get.

In a recent conversation a patient told me she was lucky if she slept thirty minutes a night, and she had been that way for many months. She was exhausted all the time and was having hormonal symptoms. Her yellow light of sleep had adequately warned her, but because she didn't know how to work on the cause, the red light of symptoms had appeared.

2. The Yellow Light of Digestion

Our digestive system is also predominantly run by the parasympathetic nervous system, and may also become out of balance when we are stressed. Symptoms may then arise. Pain, nausea, constipation, diarrhea, a "knot in the stomach", aches, and burning may all indicate a mishandling of stress. One patient I had was bothered with abdominal pains for almost forty years. As a child, her step father was very strict. He demanded absolute silence during meal time as he wanted to listen to Paul Harvey News. The stress of complying with that demand "programmed" her so that she suffered for years every time she ate. "Reprogramming" made a tremendous difference, and solved her digestive problems.

3. The Yellow Light of Healing.

The parasympathetic part of our nervous system is also responsible for healing. If that system is turned off, or down-graded as a result of emotional stress, healing may not occur.

Nicole was sixteen when she broke her leg in a horse accident. The leg was set and cast. When the doctor went to remove the cast two months later, her leg was still broken. Surgery was performed and another two months passed, and the leg still would not heal. Surgery was again performed, and a steel rod put in her leg. Two more months passed and still no healing.

That is when Nicole came to see me, wondering if we could do anything to help. I explained to Nicole that something was overriding her body's programmed ability to repair. Something in her conscious mind was overpowering the subconscious healing message to her leg, and *that* something had to be emotional. Nicole immediately knew what the cause of the stress was. She now understood how it was keeping her from healing, and she let go of the feelings she had. Her body was then able to do what it naturally knew how to do and within a month her leg was healed.

FILLING THE BOXES

We mentioned earlier that we are all born into this world with a default setting that has no fear. We call this innate default setting "child-like faith". This kind of faith allowed Brittany to happily stand erect on my hand. It allows a father to toss his son high into the air, with only giggles and laughter bubbling out of him. But experience soon teaches us to be fearful in order to survive.

If we think back to Brittany's experience on the cushion, we see that she had no reason to fear until she fell off and was hurt. Brittany's first experience with the cushion was to put it in her Safe Box, and think nothing more of it. But once she fell and was hurt, that experience with the cushion was put into her Unsafe Box. Now when she approached the edge, she cried, not wanting to repeat the hurtful experience again.

As we mature it becomes necessary to **relearn** how to have faith, if we want to overcome fear. Only this time the faith we develop is with the light on. There is a fear and faith option for each situation, and we can choose how we will respond. Choosing to have and exercise faith requires much more effort than choosing fear, but it's possible, and it's worth it.

A simple perspective of fear and faith may be useful.

§ **Faith is a belief that I, someone I trust, or God (or Higher Power) is in control.**

§ **Fear is a belief that someone or something else is in control.**

Note that belief is an important component of faith and fear. From birth to maturity we have a constant flood of experiences to put in our Boxes, so the subconscious automatically knows what to do if that experience repeats itself. There are three types of input that fill our Safe and Unsafe Boxes, with beliefs being a major factor.

1. **Survival Input** – some experiences are survival reactions to life, like any newborn animal would experience. Hunger, thirst, heat, cold, pain and injury are great teachers.

2. **Parental Input** – parents (and also siblings, friends and other authorities) train us how to act. They teach us the principles they believe and want us to believe. Animal parents also train their young how to act, but only humans teach beliefs.

3. **Our Own Input** – as we become capable to reason and

judge on our own, we choose how we perceive our experiences, and we choose what we believe.

In order to choose faith over fear, it is very helpful to understand how we became programmed the way we did, why we believe the way we do. I was talking with Lynne one day, and she told me she often felt worthless. *"Why do you think that?"* I asked. *"I've just always felt that,"* was her reply. And then she added, *"I'm just not good enough."*

Can you learn anything about what is in Lynne's Safe and Unsafe Boxes by the nature of what she said? Do you think it has any impact on her health or other aspects of her life? The idea that she was not good enough had to have been planted in stage two or three mentioned above. A baby does not come into the world with a belief that she is not good enough. It is a learned response, and therefore it can be unlearned. It had to have been a parent or other authority figure who taught her, or her own self-judgment, to cause her to have such a belief.

Lynne thought back on her life's experiences and mentioned several. As she described one, the light came on. Her step-father was an alcoholic. He was verbally and mentally abusive. At times when he had been drinking, he would drag her and her sisters out of bed in the middle of the night, sit them down at the kitchen table, and berate and belittle them. She said her sisters would cry, but she never did. She just sat there and endured it. Lynne then mentioned some things that he said, like she wasn't good enough, and that she never did anything right. That's when the light came on. That's when she realized her step-father had more of an impact on her than she thought.

Now that Lynne recognized where a thought like "not being good enough" came from, she could begin to work on changing that. What she had accepted as truth about herself was now something she could question and look at in a new light. Her ability to have faith in herself and faith that God (since she believed in God) had a greater plan for her began to increase.

Though we can't understand all the workings of faith, we can understand some of its effects in the body to cause healing. As long as we exercise faith, we are not interfering with the body's normal functions and health is the result. This is the main observation we can make. It would follow then that the more faith we are able to exert, the better our body will function and the greater its ability to heal. It is fear that interferes and leads to disease. The concept is simple, yet powerful. The application though is not so easy. How do we apply faith then to improve our health?

LETTING GO

The simplest thing we can do is to **let go**. We just need to drop the fear that we are hanging on to.

Jackie was overwhelmed. She commuted to college one hundred and sixty miles from home, returning on the weekends. She was a wife and mother of two children. Keeping up her studies, family responsibilities, and traveling was nearly impossible. Often she felt the tension of it all in her neck. Her neck would get really sore and she would develop intense headaches.

One day, when Jackie was really feeling bad, she decided to take a short break from her studies. She sat down in front of the television for a few minutes. A good movie came on which she became interested in. She thought, *"Oh well, I guess it won't hurt if I watch it."* She got totally involved in the show and forgot about everything else. When the movie ended, she realized that she felt much better. She commented, *"My neck felt fine, and my headache was completely gone."*

Jackie had solved her problem by letting go. While watching T.V., she forgot about the stresses previously plaguing her. Her body was no longer getting a fear message and so no longer reacted to the perceived threat. Her muscles relaxed and she felt fine.

Letting go is not only necessary for current stresses, but is also necessary for those in the past. Remember, all thoughts, feelings, and experiences are stored in our subconscious and are subject to immediate recall. It makes no difference when they were put in, yesterday or fifty years ago.

Lance, a truck driver, had a load of calves to haul five hundred miles. He came in for help. His back was hurting so much he wasn't sure he would be able to make the trip. He wasn't able to bend forward or turn to the right. Lance said that he had been hurting for a couple of weeks, but that it really got bad four days earlier. He had been out hunting on his horse. She stumbled and almost fell, and that's when the pain really started.

Thinking the near fall may have produced a response due to a fear of falling rather than an actual injury, I asked Lance if he had ever fallen with a horse before. He said, *"Yes, many times. In fact I've had them land on me three or four times."* I explained to him how fear of being hurt that way again could trigger a pattern from his subconscious memories, causing his pain.

I had him think about how he felt when his horse tripped. I then had him let the thought go. He was to replace it with the thought and feeling that he was grateful everything was all right, that his horse didn't fall, that the experience was over, and there was no need to fear anymore. He was lying on my treatment table and I had him move his hips and legs to send the new updated information from his mind to his muscles. When I felt his back muscles, those on the left were about fifty percent better and more relaxed than when we started.

Since our mental exercise hadn't taken care of his entire problem, I asked him when he first started having back problems. He said it was when he was in high school, almost twenty years earlier. He had been a bull rider and been thrown off and injured many times. I then had him update those memories of being hurt, let go of his fears from back then and replace them with the same positive thoughts as before. This time his back muscles melted. Now he was very relaxed. I had him stand up and bend forward. This time he could almost touch his toes. He could also turn just as far to the right as the left.

It would be nice if all health problems were that easy to solve. **Lance had no physical injury**, so there was no time needed for damaged tissue to heal. He felt fine once he let go of what he was feeling, as there was no longer a need for a fear response. It's important to recognize that the cause of his back pain began in high school, many years earlier. He had been hurt getting thrown off bulls and horses. When his horse stumbled, the memories in his Unsafe Box told him to tense up out of fear of being hurt again. A pattern for handling falling had been set, and when I saw him, he was stuck in that pattern. He was still tense, waiting to hit the ground. He needed to let go. He needed to put his near-fall experience into his Safe Box. He was able to do that, and that is why he had immediate relief.

Lance was able to let go of his fear in one session. If he did a good job of letting go of his fear of falling permanently, the next time his horse stumbled with him, he would be fine. If he only did a partial job, the fear of falling could bring the symptoms back, but at least he would understand why and know what he needed to work on.

Not all programs or patterns are that easy to change. Sometimes this change requires consistent effort over a long period of time. A one time positive thought may not replace years of negative thought. If not, then practice and repetition will always bring good results.

THE POWER OF FORGIVENESS

Sometimes letting go is not easy. Often, in order to apply our faith, we need to do a little more. We need to **forgive.**

Joan's elderly mother lived in St. Louis and needed to be moved to a nursing home. Joan's brother also lived in St. Louis, but was too busy to help. Not having any other apparent option, Joan flew eight hundred miles to assist her mother in her transition. While there, lifting a box, she strained her back.

When Joan got home she came to see me. We treated her a few times with less than desirable results. As she wasn't improving as fast as I thought she should, I explained how stress could keep her from healing. She said that she was definitely mad at her brother and considered it his fault that she had hurt her back. I told her that her body would react to anger just like any other threat and that she needed to forgive her brother. She softened as she became aware of what she was doing to herself. She was able to forgive him and in two days the back pain was gone.

That, however, was not the end of the story. Two months later Joan talked to her brother on the telephone about something else that needed to be done for their mother. Once again, her brother said he was too busy and wouldn't be able to do it. Immediately, Joan got angry and immediately, while still talking on the phone, her back began to hurt. She again came in to see me hoping that I would have an easier solution this time than forgiving her brother. I didn't. She finally concluded that she was the only one getting hurt and so there was no point hanging on to the anger. Again, she forgave her brother and once again she felt fine.

Joan's conclusion needs to be emphasized.

The only one that suffers when negative thinking is involved is the negative thinker.

Thoughts of anger and revenge only hurt the one thinking them. The best way to really get back at someone is to forgive him or her as quickly as you can. Then he or she can no longer hurt you. However, our natures are such that forgiveness is not always easy.

Ron's head was stuck to the right. He could not turn it. His wife had left him for another man and they were in the middle of an ugly divorce.

Our efforts to help Ron get well were not very successful, so I explained to him that he might have to do some forgiving. He said, *"I would rather hurt."* That was an honest, understandable answer. It was also the painful alternative, but that was his choice.

OURSELVES INCLUDED

Forgiving others is important, but forgiving ourselves may even be more important. *Sherry was depressed. The past two weeks had been especially bad. She would start crying for no apparent reason, then she didn't care about anything, and then she would suddenly burst into tears again.*

Sherry asked me to help her figure out what was wrong. As we talked, she eventually told me that a couple of weeks earlier she had a bad experience. Some pressure had been building up between her and a friend, and it had come to a head in a group situation. Sherry exploded and yelled at her friend. After doing so, she really felt bad and apologized twice. She thought the situation was taken care of, though she still felt really bad it had happened.

I asked Sherry if she continued to think about the

experience, even though she had apologized. She said she did. I explained to her that she probably hadn't forgiven herself. She couldn't let it go if she kept bringing it back up in her mind. She needed to realize that a mistake had been made, ask forgiveness, forgive herself, let it go, and learn from it. The guilt and anger she felt over her own weaknesses needed to be replaced with understanding and patience with herself. She recognized that this was what she needed to do and she did it. The gloom which hung over her was lifted. Within twenty-four hours she felt like a different person.

LOVESICK

Sometimes the kindest, most loving people we know can be the sickest. Forgiving others for them is not hard. In fact, thinking a bad thought about someone else is often very difficult. But they are not so easy on themselves. When things don't go right, they always feel that it's their fault. If their children make a wrong choice, it's because they didn't teach them right. If a spouse makes an error, it's their fault for not warning them. They tend to make everyone's problems their own. They don't like to see anyone suffer and want to do all in their power to help.

One day Melissa was in a grocery store. She saw a lady that was bald, probably from the effects of chemotherapy. Her heart really went out to this woman. Melissa wondered if she would have the nerve to go out in public if she was bald. She really felt sorry for her and thought about her often that day. About a week later, Melissa noticed that she was losing hair by the handful. It was on her pillow and everywhere.

Trying to figure out what was happening Melissa soon remembered the lady in the grocery store and realized what she was doing. She was giving up her own hair for that woman. She recognized that she had felt so much compassion for her that she had unwittingly told her subconscious to donate in an effort to solve that woman's problem. Melissa forgave herself, realizing that she couldn't solve everyone's problems, and she stopped losing her hair.

ATTITUDE OF GRATITUDE

There is a third thing we need to do to exercise faith. In

addition to letting go and forgiving, we need to **be thankful**. The old saying that "things could always be worse" is very true. So instead of concentrating on how bad they are, we need to focus on how good they are. Pain, cancer, accidents, divorce, and death all have their brighter side, if we are thankful. Our bodies react positively to gratitude since there are no perceived threats to defend against. As a result, gratitude always has a positive effect on our health.

Eileen's arthritis had flared up. She was extremely stiff in the mornings and was not sleeping well at night. She had been feeling really well and didn't know why she was now feeling worse.

I told Eileen there is always a reason for a worsening of symptoms and one she might not have thought of was stress. Eileen said that was possible as she had been "uptight" lately. Every day she went to the nursing home to visit her husband. *"I expect things to be fine, but there's always another problem,"* she said. I suggested that if she expected three problems and only found one, then it wouldn't be so stressful. She responded, *"Then I can be grateful to God that things are going so well."* I told her she was absolutely right. Her arthritis and sleep were much better as long as she was able to maintain that perspective.

We have seen how letting go, forgiving, and being thankful are the ways to relieve stress, and thus allow us to let go of the emotions which are making us unhealthy. Those three steps are mostly a mental exercise and can be done many times daily, at any time of day.

One way of applying these three principles is in sincere, heartfelt prayer, for those who believe in prayer.

Another way is when taking a walk. As you walk, determine what the fears are that are affecting you. Let go of them, forgive whoever needs to be forgiven, and express gratitude for all that you have. Often you will feel the tight muscles begin to relax right then, and you will know that you are on the right track to regain your health.

Meditation is another method to perform these positive mental exercises. One friend of mine does her morning "stretch" exercises and then spends fifteen minutes in gratitude and meditation. She thanks God for everything from the sunlight, to the flowers, to her children and husband. What a great, positive way to begin the day.

Another friend uses journaling as a way to release anger, frustration, and other emotions. He just starts writing about his feelings and anything negative that has happened. As he lets go on paper, his mood changes and he begins to see things in a more positive light. He soon is able to write about the lessons he is learning and the positive things he is experiencing.

However you choose to perform these mental exercises, you will start noticing positive results right away as you let go, forgive, and be grateful.

Let's also conclude this chapter with a summary of what we have learned.

1. **Turning on the lights:**
    a) **Allows us to see if we handle stress positively or negatively.**
    b) **Helps answer "What am I afraid of?" and "Why am I afraid?"**
    c) **Helps us recognize that we are actually choosing between faith and fear.**
2. **Indicators of how we are handling fear are:**
    a) **How we sleep.**
    b) **How we digest food.**
    c) **How we heal.**
3. **We apply faith by:**
    a) **Letting go.**
    b) **Forgiving - ourselves and others.**
    c) **Being thankful.**

Understanding and applying these concepts do much for us in our efforts to be healthy. They also go a long way in helping make life better and easier to live. They won't, however, get rid of all of life's problems. Money dilemmas, business failures, children rebelling, spouse misunderstandings, disease, and accidents will still continue to exist. What more can we do to handle the many major stresses that we live with daily?

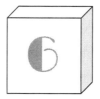

YOU BE THE JUDGE

Let's consider our Safe and Unsafe boxes again for a moment. The strongest instinct of every living being is survival. Every second of every day there are automatic processes going on that evaluate every experience, situation, and thought to determine whether we are safe or unsafe; whether everything is fine, or whether we should run or fight. That happens every moment of every day for a life time. The differences between what is found in an animal's Safe and Unsafe Boxes, and a human's are essentially these:

Animal's – determined by survival reactions.
Human's – determined by survival reactions, *and* *beliefs.*

We said in the previous chapter our Safe and Unsafe Boxes are filled by natural survival experiences, parental training and beliefs, and our own choices and beliefs. When we have an experience today, our reactions are determined by our perception of that experience compared to what was stored in the past. Said another way, we must make a judgment of every situation or experience so our body knows how to respond.

When Brittany fell off the cushion at seven months old, it was her innate survival instinct that told her the edge of the cushion was a scary place. Her mother didn't teach that to her. Experience did. It is interesting to me that later on, in the process of learning to walk, Brittany probably fell hundreds of times. She was hurt in many of those falls, yet she never sat down and refused to try walking again. Her innate intelligence was not telling her walking was wrong, just **this specific way** that caused her to fall was wrong. Learning to walk is an important life lesson and giving up on learning the lesson because we are hurt in the process is not an option.

Contrast that with Judy who was trying to heal from chronic pain and various other chronic symptoms. When something was mentioned about an experience at age six, she said, *"I'm never going back there! That was too painful!"* Whatever it was that happened to Judy at age six, she didn't want to ever think about it or talk about it again.

What is Judy saying? Isn't it likely she is refusing to learn some important life lesson because the pain is too great? Isn't there likely still some important lesson for her to learn that could even help her today? The experiences, and emotions from those experiences, ideally would be brought into the light and dealt with somehow. Figuratively, we could say the pain from falling at age six is keeping her from learning to walk.

At some point, Judy went from an infant willing to risk all kinds of hurt and injury in order to walk, to a child unwilling to learn an important life lesson because of the pain. Most of us have done the same. What happened to Judy that caused her to falter in her progress? She began to reason.

THE SEASON TO REASON
We as human beings have the gift of choice that allows us to think and reason. It seems to be a gift that grows with us. Thankfully it develops slowly. Our desire to learn to walk at age one greatly outweighs the danger of trying. If the ability to reason came at age one, we may have decided the falls weren't worth the effort, and may have never learned to walk or run.

Renee recalled a vivid memory at about age four. Her father was rather abusive at times, and she remembered him getting mad at her one year old sister one day and throwing her against the wall. She remembered thinking that was a wrong thing to do.

Renee's Unsafe Box contained enough information in it at age four that she could reason and make a judgment. The judgment she made was that the thing her dad had done was wrong. Renee's parents and others had been teaching her some basics of what was right and wrong, and she was now able to compare her sister's experience to the beliefs she had learned. Those beliefs allowed her to make a judgment that dad had done a bad thing.

What about Renee's little sister? She was too young to have the reasoning capacity of Renee, so she could not judge it as Renee did. Her reaction would be more like an animal that also cannot reason, yet can be trained. She was physically hurt, so her survival instinct would put memories in her Unsafe Box about her dad which could cause her to react differently to him than before. She could feel unsafe around him as she matured, but none of that would be conscious. Any reaction she might have would be due to subconscious survival training.

Renee had enough beliefs stored in her Safe and Unsafe Box that she was able to reason between good and bad, and right and wrong, and as a result, make a judgment. Judy had done the same thing with what happened to her at age six. We all don't have the same survival experiences and beliefs stored in our Boxes. That's one reason we are all so unique and don't all see things the same way.

Suppose Renee's dad changed his ways after the above incident and spent the rest of his life being a loving, caring father. Could Renee's perception of her dad change, and cause her to react differently to him than she would otherwise? Could she think and reason again, and put him in her Safe Box? Of course she could, but it may take a long time with much forgiveness. Her ability to reason is the gift that would allow her to make the change.

TWO WAYS TO JUDGE

Our ability to choose allows us to reason and make judgment. As we mature our ability to reason and make judgment increases. It is important to note that there are two ways a judgment is made.

1. **Automatic – based on what we have learned in the past. Requires no thought.**
   a. **Can be Physical**
   b. **Can be Emotional**

2. **Willful Choice – based on reason, logic, and agency. Requires thought.**
   a. **Can be Physical**
   b. **Can be Emotional**

A *physical automatic judgment* is our fight or flight survival response, such as when a bear comes into the room. It is easy to understand why that reaction is necessary, for our very life is being threatened.

An *emotional automatic reaction* is just as real, though not as readily understood. Chad gets chest pain when he becomes overwhelmed. Martha eats a sandwich when she thinks someone is attracted to her. They experience automatic reactions just as real as if a bear entered the room, but those reactions are based on **more** than physical survival. Those reactions involve emotional survival which is based on past emotional experiences and how those experiences were handled according to Martha and Chad's feelings and beliefs. Both physical and emotional automatic judgments produce a programmed reaction in our body according to our perceived need. Depending on whether we automatically solve the problem or are holding on to the emotions the problem presents, we may or may not like the outcome. Escaping the bear and not becoming his lunch is wonderful; frequent episodes of chest pain are not.

The second way we make a judgment is *willful choice*. This too involves physical and emotional survival. When we see that the bear in the room is our pet bear Teddy, we consciously reason that we are safe and that there is no need to run. We think it through. We look at the thing threatening us and use our agency to decide how to respond. When Chad came to understand the cause of his chest pain, he could apply reason and logic to willfully see it differently. He was then free to make a choice that allowed him to respond in a different way so chest pain was unnecessary. Judy judged that her experience at six years old was so bad that she would never revisit it. That too is a willful choice, and one that can be changed.

THE TWO JUDGMENTS

There are two ways to judge an experience or situation, and there are two types of judgment we make.

1. **Initial Judgment**
2. **Final Judgment**

The Initial Judgment, whether it is automatic or chosen, determines our body's reaction to that experience. We then store that experience in our Safe Box or Unsafe Box, depending on how we judged it.

The Final Judgment is where we choose in which box to leave that experience. We don't have to keep it in the same box we initially put it in, though we may. The Final Judgment may happen by default, meaning the Initial Judgment becomes the Final Judgment because we never question it. The Final Judgment may also happen by reason and thought and we consciously decide in which box that experience is to stay.

Wayne came in because he was having headaches. The only time he had headaches though, was when he rode in a car. If he drove for fifty miles, he would have a migraine that would put him in bed for a day.

Would it make sense that Wayne had some kind of mental or emotional programming going on that resulted in his migraines? Wayne had been in four car accidents. Wayne had stored the experience of riding in a car in his Unsafe Box. He knew that accident number five was just over the hill or waiting just around the corner, and survival reactions accompanied him accordingly. In order to get rid of his headaches, Wayne needed to move his accident memories from his Unsafe Box to his Safe Box. He was able to do that by recognizing that the accidents could have been a lot worse and being grateful that they weren't. He was grateful for the safety and protection he had received and was truly able to feel that gratitude.

Wayne's Initial Judgment of his car accidents was to put

them in his Unsafe Box. That is natural and spontaneous when one's life is physically threatened. If his Final Judgment had been to keep them there, he would have had headaches each time he rode in a car for the rest of his life. He understood what he was doing to himself, used letting go, faith and gratitude, and decided that his Final Judgment would be to put them in his Safe Box. As a result he had no more headaches when traveling. Eventually he was able to enjoy a two thousand mile road trip without a headache.

THE LAW OF WITNESSES

It is important to note here that the first judgment is both an Initial Judgment and a Final Judgment. It is spontaneous and without thought. The experience is either safe or unsafe, and we respond automatically. We have no reason to see it differently. Wayne's first auto accident would have been stored in his Unsafe Box. That's where it should be stored as he was injured. That was his Initial and Final judgment of the car accident at that time.

But he could get in a car after that first accident and drive as far as he wanted, without having headaches. Yet, after he had his second accident, something changed dramatically in him. This is what is called the *Law of Witnesses*. It often seems that the first time we have an experience as Wayne did, we can perceive it as random, or by chance. The likelihood of it happening again isn't really considered. But after it happens a second time, it is no longer perceived as a random or chance thing. It is perceived as reality and serves as a warning that we had better be careful. If it happened twice, it easily could happen a third time. We may now begin to live in fear of that thing, and physical symptoms may start to appear.

In a court of law, the testimony of two or more witnesses that corroborate each other strengthens the case. Wayne might say that the testimony of two accidents is true as well. Four accidents, or four testimonies, are so powerful that a fifth accident must be considered imminent. How could it not be? Wayne has the experiences that tell him that accidents are his reality. The beauty of the conscious mind is that we do have a choice to see things differently.

Let's see how this worked with one more accident victim.

Rosemary was in an accident where she had rolled her vehicle. She came to our office because her neck was hurting.

We treated Rosemary and she got better. Six months later she came to our office again, not being able to turn her head because of neck pain. She had been driving down the road when she had a blow-out on a rear tire of her car. She said her neck immediately tightened up as she slowly pulled her car off to the side of the road. Interestingly, there were four other people in the car, and she was the only one who got a stiff neck.

Though Rosemary was not in an accident, her memory of her previous accident six months earlier was immediately recalled. It was enough of a second witness to remind her of her first accident and the result was a stiff neck.

Here is a great secret to healing and wellness:

Take all memories, thoughts and feelings out of the Unsafe Box and put them in the Safe Box.

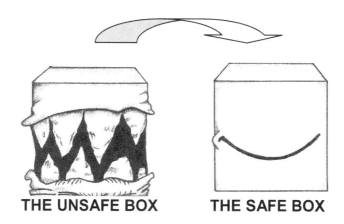

THE UNSAFE BOX   **THE SAFE BOX**

This is one of the most important concepts you will read in this book. It is one of the *3 Steps to Heal Yourself* that we will expound on in Part 2. It can be relatively easy, or take a lot of work, depending on you. This book is written to help you realize it is possible, and to make that change.

Any memory stored in our Unsafe Box has some degree of effect on us physically. The number of memories stored, and how negatively we feel about them, determine the type and degree of symptoms. You might think of your symptoms as a measuring stick or thermometer. As you transfer memories from your Unsafe Box to your Safe Box, you should see your thermometer of symptoms go down.

Rhonda said she had become gluten intolerant and hadn't been able to eat wheat for fifteen years. However, she had been able to eat wheat the first forty years of her life.

Of course that brought a question to my mind. What happened fifteen years earlier? It took Rhonda a while to remember, and then it dawned on her. She had been walking to the bakery to buy bread when she got bit by a dog. She had to get a rabies shot, which she didn't want to do. She was in a foreign country and there was three months of confrontational issues with the dog owners and the government before it was all resolved. Can you see how Rhonda's Initial Judgment of this experience caused bread to end up in her Unsafe Box? Every time she had bread after that, her stomach would knot up, and digestion would shut down. The bread, or even the thought of eating bread, put her into a fight or flight response. She diagnosed herself as gluten intolerant and quit eating wheat products. She worked through that memory, and made a Final Judgment to store it in her Safe Box. She started eating a little bit of wheat, didn't have a reaction and doesn't have a problem with wheat today.

John had an allergy to cats. His eyes would water, his nose would run, and he would break out into an irritating rash when he walked into a room where a cat had been.

John said he grew up with cats, and didn't react to the ones his family had, just those belonging to someone else. When I explained how he might be reacting to a negative memory with cats, he recalled what had happened. He was four years old and his family was on its way home from getting their first cat when it *"about bit my thumb off"*. From what John said, it would appear that he stored cat experiences in each of the boxes. In the Safe Box were cats he knew he could trust. In the Unsafe Box were those he wasn't so sure about. Once John was able to make a Final Judgment on his memory at four years old and store it in his Safe Box, the thermometer of his symptoms gradually diminished. A month later he didn't have any more allergic reactions to cats, and still didn't when I talked to him a year later.

PROPER JUDGMENT

You will notice as we have talked about judging, we have talked about judging situations and experiences. We have not talked about judging people. Dallin Oaks gave some wise counsel on this matter.

"Whenever possible we will refrain from judging people and only judge situations." (Dallin H. Oaks, "'Judge Not' and Judging", *Ensign,* Aug 1999, 7)

This can be a hard lesson to learn, especially when we have been a victim. In the same article, Oaks quotes the words of a victim of childhood sexual abuse. She too has made tremendous progress in her life, and learned some extremely valuable lessons.

"I am a survivor of childhood physical, emotional, and sexual abuse. I no longer view myself as a victim. The change has come from inside me – my attitude. I do not need to destroy myself with anger and hate. I don't need to entertain thoughts of revenge… I am responsible for my actions and what I do with my knowledge. I am not to blame for what happed to me as a child. I cannot change the past. But I can change the future. I have chosen to heal myself and pass on to my children what I have learned. The ripples in my pond will spread through future generations." (Dallin H. Oaks, "'Judge Not' and Judging", *Ensign,* Aug 1999, 7)

This woman's life-changing attitude reminds me of a favorite quote by Charles Swindoll.

"The longer I live, the more I realize the impact of attitude on life. Attitude, to me, is more important than facts. It is more important than the past, than education, than money, than circumstances, than failures, than successes, than what other people think or say or do. It is more important than appearance, giftedness, or skill. It will make or break a company…a church…a home. The remarkable thing is we have a choice every day regarding the attitude we will embrace for that day. We cannot change our past…we cannot change the fact that people

will act in a certain way. We cannot change the inevitable. The only thing we can do is play on the one thing we have, and that is our attitude... I am convinced that life is 10% what happens to me and 90% how I react to it." (http://www.famous-quotes.com/author.php?aid=7098)

THE TIME TO HEAL

When the cause is identified, and the attitude is redirected, amazing things happen. Many symptoms can disappear quickly. Relief is immediate, and the body rapidly recovers. In such cases there is no need for the body to repair or rebuild.

June suffered with constipation for four years. She only had a bowel movement every four or five days and only then if she took a laxative.

It all started when June's husband got sick and she became a care giver. He lived a year and then passed away. If we are emotionally hanging on, not wanting to let go, the emotion may manifest itself physically as constipation. I explained this to June, and suggested this was the pattern she was stuck in. She was in the process of selling their farm and making lots of changes in her life. She knew she needed to let go, and this was a good time to do it. She went home with a resolve to work on it. I talked to her a week later. She'd had three bowel movements the day after I saw her and was back to her regular routine of a bowel movement every day.

In June's case, there was nothing for the body to heal or repair. It only needed a different message in order to respond differently. Some symptoms can be cleared up quickly like this, but some conditions, especially chronic degenerative conditions, can take a long time for the body to rebuild and improve. There are often many layers of "stuff" to work through. Fixing one memory may not do much symptomatically if there are a hundred more to go. But it is a start, and a place to begin. Improving your diet is often another necessary step for healing and repairing of chronic degenerative conditions.

So far in this book we have focused mainly on symptomatic relief. Some health problems may initially have very few symptoms associated with them. Bone loss, plaque build up in the arteries, and tumor growth are a few examples of conditions that may slowly and quietly develop without a person's awareness. Thus it becomes important to not just focus on symptoms, but on wellness. Choosing a healthy lifestyle will do much to prevent the chronic degenerative types of disease. Wellness is a lifetime project.

Roxanne had been told that she would need cataract surgery in a year. The year had passed so she went back to the doctor to see what would need to be done. To his surprise and hers, she no longer had a cataract, and her field of vision had improved significantly. Her eyes were better than they had been in several years. She gave credit to the fact that she had improved her diet, taken some good supplements, and worked on the emotional things that "kept her from seeing".

People recover, heal and repair from all kinds of conditions, major or minor, using the same approach as Roxanne. People stay healthy and well for the same reason. The body is remarkable. There is nothing more amazing or wonderful on this earth.

THE LAWS OF HEALING AND WELLNESS

As I have worked in the health and wellness field for over thirty years, and have pondered on various lessons and observations, I have discovered four laws that govern healing and wellness. They resonate as truth with me, and are the foundation of what I believe and practice. The first law is:

The body never makes a mistake. It does everything it does for a reason.

This First Law has been the major focus of the book to this point. You should have a better understanding and appreciation of that fact now, than when you first opened the cover. The next three chapters will discuss the remaining three laws, and the impact they have on your health and wellness.

The Four Laws are as follows:

THE 4 LAWS OF HEALING AND WELLNESS

1. **The body never makes a mistake. Everything it does is for a reason.**
2. **Correct Emotional Choices lead to healing and wellness.**
3. **Correct Nutritional Choices lead to healing and wellness.**
4. **Correct Physical Choices lead to healing and wellness.**

My intent in this book is to show that these Four Laws are interrelated and are true. I want to give the reader explanations of them and tools to apply them. Symptoms we experience, especially chronic symptoms, are indicators we are not following these laws. Applying each of these laws will always lead to better health.

Let's summarize what we have learned in this chapter.

1. **A judgment is made two ways – automatically and by willful choice.**
2. **There are two types of judgments – Initial and Final.**
3. **A great secret to healing is: take memories, thoughts and feelings out of the Unsafe Box and put them in the Safe Box.**
4. **Refrain from judging people, only judge situations.**
5. **Understand and apply the Laws of Healing and Wellness.**

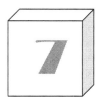

THE EMOTIONAL SAFE BOX

Tom had high blood pressure and digestive problems for years. He wanted to try something more natural than what he was doing so he came into our office.

As we began to explain these healing concepts to Tom, he was amazed. He was a well read man and very intelligent, but had made no connection between his physical symptoms and the stresses that he had experienced in his life. This was all new territory for him, but it made a lot of sense. He knew that his struggles with a couple of his children had affected him emotionally, but he didn't understand the physical connection. He didn't realize how his reactions to these experiences had affected his health, but it was clicking with him now. He told me later that as he drove the forty miles home, insights and enlightenment came to him as memories popped into his head. It was truly an epiphany for him, and he felt *"weight after weight"* leaving his body. He literally had a change of heart. And as happens each time, his symptoms began to change as well.

EMOTIONAL PROTECTION

As we grow up and experience life, we soon learn that we will be emotionally hurt. We learn that people in whom we automatically put our trust will eventually do things that hurt us in some way. It is just what happens in life. And thus, we learn the importance of emotionally protecting ourselves.

Harold was about fifty years old, and had digestive problems most of his life. It was normal for him to have twelve or thirteen bowel movements a day. A good day was only five or six. He remembered having stomach aches as a young child and going to the doctor often and even spending time in the hospital. The only diagnosis he remembers being given was "stress".

If we look to the chart in Chapter 3 that shows the body's reaction to stress, it says under Digestion:

System of the Body	1. The Immediate Reaction	2. The Long Term Reaction	3. Eventual Possible Chronic Conditions
Digestion	Slows down (need to run or fight, not digest)	Poor digestion, deficiency of acid and enzymes	Acid reflux, constipation, hiatal hernia

Stress could undoubtedly be the reason for Harold's excessive number of trips to the bathroom; so could memories from long ago that caused such a condition to be "normal". His body had to eliminate so he could deal with the bear that was chasing him. Harold also said that fatigue was a major complaint, and he had a hard time making it through a day without taking something stimulating. Can you see why? Who wouldn't be tired after running from a bear for so many years? In addition, what kind of nutrition was he actually getting out of his food if it traveled through his digestive tract so quickly? He also commented that he was hungry all the time – not surprising.

I asked Harold if he could come up with any early childhood memories of things that had been fairly stressful or frightening for him. He came up with two. They happened when he was five years old.

Harold said the first day of kindergarten was awful. He wanted his mom to take him, but she just showed him where the bus stop was and made him ride the bus. It was a very frightening experience. All the other kids were with their moms at kindergarten, and he wondered why his mom hadn't come with him.

The second experience happened during story time in

kindergarten. Harold said his teacher was old and mean, and that he was very afraid of her. He didn't want to do anything to make her angry because she would yell and even spank the kids. He was sitting in his desk listening to the story, running his finger along the molding of the desk. Suddenly his teacher slammed her ruler on the desk and yelled at him for not paying attention. Harold remembered his exact thoughts, *"I told Mom this lady was mean. She should have listened to me and not made me come to kindergarten!"*

Each of these experiences was very vivid and real to Harold. He could remember them like they happened yesterday. He remembered his exact thoughts, the exact words that were said, and the feelings he had. He also realized, for the first time, that they were related to Mom.

Harold had been emotionally hurt. He had expected protection and safety from his mother, as that is what he had always experienced. That was his automatic default setting with which he had been born into the world, an automatic default setting that all was well and safe. There was no reason to fear emotionally as he had never been hurt emotionally. But now he had been hurt, and by the one he knew loved him the most. How could that be?

A better question might be, how could it not be? Harold's mom undoubtedly did what she thought was best for her son by sending him off to kindergarten on his own. What if she had taken him to kindergarten the first day? Would she have had to take him the second day as well? At what point would Harold feel safe enough in that class, with that mean old lady, to tell his mom he didn't need her anymore?

Harold experienced something that all of us experience, and that is emotional hurt. It is a necessary part of life, just as necessary as physical pain to learn life's lessons. Harold's innate expectation that his mother would protect him had to end somewhere. It could not go on forever. Harold could not always live under Mom's protective wing. He must eventually learn to fly himself. Mom and dad wanted him to learn, and so may have pushed him into circumstances that he may not have felt were safe.

The inborn automatic faith and trust we have in our

parents must eventually be replaced with faith and trust by choice. We must forgive and let go of any hurt they may have caused, no matter how hurtful it was. We must put them in our Safe Box.

Harold could see from these memories that he had some work to do. They were emotionally painful when he thought of them. He made a statement, a type of which I hear frequently, *"Having my kindergarten teacher yell at me shouldn't be a traumatic memory in my fifties!"*

Had Harold touched a hot stove at age five and been burned physically, he would not suddenly think that it was now okay at age fifty to touch a hot stove. Being "burned" emotionally is not really any different than being burned physically. It is painful and something we do not want to repeat. Those memories were still in his Unsafe Box, or he would not have felt so emotional when he thought of them. His Final Judgment of his kindergarten experiences was still the same as his Initial Judgment. They were still unsafe. If he wanted to feel differently about them, and especially if he wanted to get over his digestive issues, he needed to make a new Final Judgment of those experiences and put them in his Safe Box, and leave them there. He certainly could do that. That is the beauty of willful choice and the magnificent mind we have been given!

VIVID LESSONS

Harold's story brings up an important point. As he reflected back on those memories at age five, they were very vivid and real to him. He could remember the exact words said and his exact thoughts. He could see exactly where he was and what he was doing, all in living, vibrant color as if it were yesterday. Renee had the same vivid memory of her sister being thrown against the wall, recalling each specific word she thought. The important lesson to note is:

In the vivid memory are emotions to be dealt with and lessons to be learned.

Vivid memories like the ones Harold and Renee recalled are sitting there with a spotlight shining on them, begging to be resolved. You will remember Judy, the one who didn't want to revisit her memories from age six. She had a spotlight shining on hers as well. She just didn't yet know how to look without being afraid. If it takes fifty years or more, learning the lessons from our vivid memories will still have a significant effect on us, spiritually, emotionally, and physically.

Of course not all memories from which we can learn are so vivid. Some are faint or vague. Others are deeply buried and long forgotten. These too may also have something to teach us. In Part 2 we will share more specific ideas on how to learn from these other types of memories.

TRUSTING GOD

We defined faith earlier as a belief that *I, someone I trust, or God (or Higher Power) is in control of a situation.* If we naturally begin to have less trust and confidence in our parents and others in authority over us, because of physical and emotional hurts, what about our relationship with God? Is a belief in God necessary for good health?

For some people, God is the ultimate Safe Box. Picturing God's hand in every experience of life creates a wonderful sense of safety and well-being. For others, a belief in God could be the ultimate Unsafe Box. Seeing his hand in every experience can range from nonsense to extreme fear. It all depends on one's beliefs.

We don't have to look very hard to see that faith and trust in God is generally questioned as we mature. By the time a child reaches his teenage years, he's had enough experience to question just about everything. This is a good and necessary step, for faith and trust in God is a choice to be made, not a belief to be enforced. For most people that trust is natural and innate at birth, questioned with time and experience, and decided upon with time and experience.

So if we believe in God, what is his role in our health? How much say does he have in it? How much does he get involved?

Wendy was dealing with cancer for the third time, this time cancer of the colon. It all began ten years earlier when she was diagnosed with cancer of the gall bladder. She described herself as a very pious person at the time, praying five times a day, and having a wonderful relationship with God. Then she received the cancer diagnosis.

"Why?" she asked herself. *"Why did God allow this to happen to me? What am I doing wrong?"* Several more tests followed, and the results came back – she did not have cancer. Her gall bladder was inflamed, that was all. What would your reaction be if you were Wendy? Happy? Relieved? Ecstatic? Wendy's was one of anger. *"Why would God play this cruel trick on me?"* were her words.

Was God playing a trick? Did He give her cancer, or take it away, or have anything to do with it? Did her subsequent experiences with cancer have anything to do with God playing a trick?

If Wendy had come into my office with her complaint of gall bladder problems, my office manager, Dottie, would have had a suggestion for her. When Dottie came to work for me, she'd had gall bladder problems for several months. In fact she was scheduled to have her gall bladder removed in two weeks. Dottie would have told Wendy that a few dietary changes had made all the difference, and she never did have her gall bladder removed. (See Chapter 8 for more information on nutrition.) She would have told Wendy there was a natural solution, and she likely would not need to have her gall bladder removed. Knowing Dottie, she also would have told Wendy it was her diet, not God that was playing tricks on her.

THE CHANGING BODY

It is important to remember again that there is nothing better or grander on the earth than the human body. It is marvelous in its design and amazing in its function. From the moment of conception, a chain of events is set in place to create a self-regenerating, self-healing body.

Consider how your body changes. You really are not the same person you were last year. Did you know the body replaces the lining of the stomach about every five days, the skin about every thirty days, the liver about every six weeks, the skeleton about every three months, and the red blood cells about every four months? Your body is constantly renewing itself. Much of what the body does is like being on automatic pilot. It's what we do today that affects the body we have tomorrow, not what God does, or whether or not God exists. An animal does not need to believe in God to be healthy and neither do we. Our health is determined by the food we eat, the beverages we drink, the quality of air we breathe, the exercise and rest we get or don't get, and most importantly, the stress we feel and how we respond to it. As Dottie would say, there is no point in blaming God for tricking us. We have plenty of opportunities to do that to ourselves.

GOD DIDN'T DESERT YOU!

Maya had one child and wanted another. She'd had four miscarriages since her baby had been born, and came to see if I had some nutritional or other suggestions for her that might help.

I treated Maya, gave her some nutritional recommendations, and expected that the next time she got pregnant, the results would be different. They weren't. Maya got pregnant, and once again had a miscarriage. I suggested to Maya that we were missing something. She then told me the rest of the story.

Maya had gone off to college after high school. The week before classes started she went to a barbecue about thirty miles out of town. As the gathering dispersed at the end of the party, a young man she thought she could trust offered to give her a ride home. On the way back to town he stopped the car and became forceful. He did some very inappropriate things. Maya wasn't raped, but it was close. Maya was victimized and violated. *"I can't be pregnant!"* was one of the thoughts that ran forcefully through her mind.

When you know the rest of the story, it is easy to see why Maya couldn't stay pregnant and would miscarry. She had told herself she couldn't be pregnant, and she meant it! There were some unresolved emotions from her traumatic experience that were still affecting her. In fact her first pregnancy had been very difficult, and she and her husband feared she would lose the baby many times. She spent most of the pregnancy in bed and on medication so she wouldn't lose the baby. She had other symptoms as well. For several years she had suffered from severe back pain and a very irregular menstrual cycle.

Maya wondered why God had deserted her. Here she was, off to college doing what she should, and God allowed this to happen. Why? Why did he desert her? Why did He abandon her?

Maya believed in God just like Wendy, and just like Wendy, Maya had placed God in her Unsafe Box. I said to Maya, *"God didn't desert you. He was with you. He protected you. It could have been worse. You weren't raped."*

Maya looked at me astonished, and then replied, *"I hadn't looked at it like that!"* That thought changed her. It made a lot of sense to her, and she suddenly began to see the whole experience differently. She began to truly grasp what God protecting her meant. It was a complete and sudden 180 degree shift in perspective. In so doing, she moved God and her experience from the Unsafe Box to the Safe Box.

Maya awoke the next morning without any back pain, the first time in three years. She was able to just lie in bed and relax. Previously, the pain in her back had been so intense every morning, she would have to crawl out of bed and crawl to the dresser to pull herself up. Soon Maya was pregnant and had a regular, normal pregnancy.

There is a great lesson to be learned here. When Maya could see God's protective hand in her life, she was safe. Her unsafe experience all of a sudden became a safe experience. One of the most powerful ways to move something from our Unsafe Box into our Safe Box is to know God was there with us through every moment of that experience. It is a matter of choice to see it that way, and it may require a change of belief. Sometimes, as the familiar *Footprints in the Sand* poem tells us, God carries us. We may think we are walking the path alone, but we never are. A powerful phrase of trust and faith we can tell ourselves in any circumstance or situation is:

I'm grateful God protected me and guided me through this.

That phrase worked for Maya. It works for all of us who

choose to believe in God. It is a powerful way to see God's hand in our lives. When we can do that, we feel safe, and our physical body has no reason to exercise survival reactions.

The world we live in is full of good and bad. There are many variables that make life interesting and give us an environment in which we can learn and grow. When people choose to act in a bad way, God is not to blame. The right of free choice allows us all to act as well as react. When someone uses this gift to hurt us, we may feel that God has "allowed" it, and therefore is to blame. That perspective is also a choice. A better and safer choice is to remember that though he allows it, he is there for us, even in the worst of circumstances.

To change our thoughts and feelings about our current situations and past experiences is not easy. But what is often even more difficult is leaving them in our Safe Box once we have made the change. In reality it is fairly easy to forgive and let go in the moment. It is the reminders that come up in thousands of different ways that cause us to undo our good intentions and change our Final Judgment. Then back to the Unsafe Box we go, with its attending ailments.

TWO REASONS

There are two major reasons why it is difficult to keep experiences in our Safe Box, and improve. Let me illustrate by telling you about Carla.

Carla had an eating disorder for several years. She had been to doctors and counselors and had shown little improvement. She had discussed much with them about the problems in her life, and why she was the way she was, but to no avail. Her eating disorder continued.

Carla's illness persisted because she had not identified and fixed the **cause** of her behavior. After visiting with her and hearing her story, I explained that I thought she needed to forgive her ex-husband in order to get well. She worked on that with little success. At times she was somewhat forgiving, but at other times, very resentful and bitter.

It also became apparent that Carla had another problem. In an effort to help her forgive, and knowing she had a religious background, I asked her if she prayed. She said she used to, but not anymore. After months and months of fervent and pleading prayer that God would change her husband and preserve their marriage, divorce became imminent. She had lost faith in God and began to believe he was not interested in her life. Her desire for prayer ceased as she attempted to handle life on her own. Carla could not get well for two reasons.

1. She had not identified the correct cause of her problem.

Though it is not always necessary to identify all the stresses that have lead to a person's illness, it is important to recognize the major ones. A major cause of Carla's problem was she would no longer trust anyone close to her, not even God. She was living in fear. She needed to forgive and put God back into her life. Because she believed in God, she couldn't just say he did not exist, so she had put him in her Unsafe Box. She didn't trust him. It was impossible for her to feel safe and be healthy as a result. Carla was willing to start praying again when I suggested she not ask for anything, but just express gratitude. This was a big step toward being able to overcome reason number two.

2. She kept taking back what she had let go of.

Carla had never been completely able to forgive her husband. She could half-heartedly do it for a little while, but when the money was scarce, or her children needed a dad, the anger came back. Her experiences with him continued to reside in her Unsafe Box, and as a result, she had not yet been able to get well.

Like Carla, if we are not feeling as if we are progressing, then we either have not identified our problems correctly, or we are not truly letting go. Let's take a closer look at these two possibilities.

PROPER IDENTIFICATION

First, how do we correctly identify what is interfering?

Phyllis had chronic low back pain. She was very

overweight, though she had been on "every diet in the world". When she returned to a normal eating pattern, she would quickly put back on the weight she had lost, and more.

Phyllis and I talked about how her condition might be more of an emotional problem than a nutritional, chemical, or physical one. I explained to her how our physical bodies often reflect what is in our minds, and maybe she was carrying lots of emotional baggage. She recalled that she had not had a weight problem until, as a child, she moved to a neighborhood she did not like. She felt rejected there and so she ate to compensate. She specifically remembered sitting at the kitchen table eating all the sandwiches on the plate so the kids outside wouldn't get any. This was a very vivid memory. Phyllis was able to rethink that memory and put it in her Safe Box. She was able to forgive the other kids, and herself for how she reacted to them, and let go of that rejection.

Did that resolve her weight problem? No. That was just the beginning. Phyllis began to realize she had a lot of emotional "garbage" buried within her that she needed to get rid of. She had never considered this before. She knew she couldn't clear all of it out on her own, and that she needed help. The one who knew her best was God, and she turned to him for answers. Experiences, many long since forgotten, but inappropriately handled, came to mind. Thoughts and feelings were released and Phyllis became a new woman inside. No matter how big or little the event, she was able to give it up. She knew she had to make every memory safe, or she couldn't get well. It was not an easy process, but it was a very rewarding one. She came to know that God really was there for her, and she understood how much she could depend on him.

Phyllis was also able to share some of her feelings with a close and trusted friend. She also used some of the techniques described in Part 2 of this book. These were all very helpful in her healing process. She lost weight and continues to lose weight today.

CUTTING WHEELS

The second reason we might not be successful at properly identifying the cause of our problems, is our inability to completely let go. We often keep taking things back.

One day my daughter, who was two years old at the time, cut her finger with her mother's cutting wheel, a small hand tool she used for sewing. After a little extra love, time, and of course a Band-Aid, it was healed. A week later, my wife, Debi, was using the cutting wheel again. Jessica saw the wheel, looked at her finger, and immediately began to cry. Debi was at first amused with her response. Jessica cried and complained until my wife finally believed her finger actually did hurt, and put another Band-Aid on it.

What happened? Simply seeing the cutting wheel was enough to bring Jessica's negative experience back to reality, and the hurt along with it. She hadn't yet let go of the first frightening experience. In her mind, she might as well have been cut again.

Carla had a similar experience. She understood that she needed to forgive her ex-husband for the things he had put her through, but reality made it difficult. The emotional scars were extremely deep, and the difficult challenges of life were easily blamed on him. She attempted forgiveness, often sincerely, but then another "cutting wheel" would show itself and the hurt would start all over. Carla was not able to let go.

In order to let go, Carla needed to see things differently. The light needed to be turned on. Something needed to happen so she could see things differently. The answer for Carla came when she decided to truly exercise faith in her beliefs about God and his role in her life, instead of focusing on the hurts and wrongs caused by her ex-husband. She literally began to believe what she believed. That extra effort made the difference. To truly believe in what you believe can be very healing.

FORGIVING SELF

Annette had one or two migraines a month. We had treated her many times but she improved very little. We helped her change her diet and worked on many emotional stresses, yet she still didn't get the anticipated improvements.

One day Annette said to me, *"I watched television yesterday and was feeling really good. Then a program came on about the family. I soon noticed I had a migraine and thought it must be because of something said in the program. I think the trigger to my migraines is when I wish I had been a better mom."*

Could such a thought trigger migraines? Of course it could. Then Annette told me through tear filled eyes how she wasn't as good a mother as she should have been. We talked about forgiveness, and especially her being able to forgive herself.Personal application of forgiveness can be difficult for even the best of people. We have a hard time forgiving ourselves since we knew better, or know we should have done better. Yet if we want to get well, it is one of the most powerful things we can do.

Boyd Packer shared this wonderful analogy of self forgiveness, *"So many live with accusing guilt when relief is ever at hand. So many are like the immigrant woman who skimped and saved and deprived herself until, by selling all of her possessions, she bought a steerage-class ticket to America. She rationed out the meager provisions she was able to bring with her. Even so, they were gone early in the voyage. When others went for their meals, she stayed below deck—determined to suffer through it. Finally, on the last day, she must, she thought, afford one meal to give her strength for the journey yet ahead. When she asked what the meal would cost, she was told that all of the meals had been included in the price of her ticket."* (Boyd K. Packer, "The Brilliant Morning of Forgiveness," *New Era*, Apr 2005, 4)

Like the immigrant woman, Annette's relief is literally ever at hand. By letting go and forgiving herself, her migraines would no longer exist. There could even be other aspects of her life that would improve as well.

THINK ABOUT WHAT YOU THINK ABOUT

If you pay attention to the thoughts in your head, to your mental conversations, you will notice you often bounce back and forth between what you think and what you think others think. Pay special attention to your feelings and your body's reactions as you do so. Do your shoulders tense up? Does your stomach feel upset? Do you notice any emotional or physical reaction to your mental conversations?

As you try to keep yourself in the Safe Box, it is important to:

1. **Think about what you think about.**
2. **Think about what you think others think about.**

Andrea's neck, shoulder and arm pain started a month earlier when she was running on the tread mill. It was continuing to get worse and was aggravated by exercising.

We would expect a physical injury to be improving over time, not getting worse. I talked to Andrea about stress, and how it may be keeping her from healing. We treated her a few times, each time dealing with some stress or past memories. Overall she was improving, but there were times when her neck would really tighten up. Then we had a discussion about "thinking about what you think about", and "thinking about what you think others are thinking about".

Andrea came in the next visit saying her neck was much better, with barely any stiffness. She said, *"Thinking about what I am thinking about has really made a difference. When my neck starts to stiffen up, I ask myself, what am I thinking about? Each time I find I am irritated about something. They are different things, but I am always feeling irritated. I then can let it go and feel my neck and shoulder relax."*

AM I DONE YET?

How do we know when we have accomplished our task? How do we know when we have identified all the problems, forgiven others and ourselves, let go of what we need to, and are thinking correctly?

Braden had a problem with putting himself down. He felt he was never quite as good as anyone else, and others always seemed to have it better than him. There was always a "But if only ..." ready to come out of his mouth. If he was only as smart as John, or as talented as Bill, he would have it made. At times these comparisons would lead him into periods of depression. He would eventually come out of them, but there was always a negative feeling hanging over him. He said he occasionally wished someone would find a brain tumor, and then he would at least have an explanation for the way he was. He thought that would even be a relief.

Braden and I talked a few times and he was very willing to try the things I suggested. He identified some of the problems in his life, and concentrated on the forgiveness and letting go which was necessary. But he was still having too many days where he didn't feel right and just wanted to give up.

Finally I asked him if he was grateful for this trial in his life. He said, *"What?"* I asked him again if he was thankful for the experiences of the past forty years. He said he wasn't and asked what I meant. I told him we are to learn from the experiences we have in life. They are our teachers and we should be grateful for the lessons they teach us.

I explained that if he wasn't thankful for lessons learned, then he hadn't yet learned what he needed to from them. He would continue to have these negative feelings until he could appreciate the learning experience they presented. Then there would be no need for them anymore. This thought clicked with Braden and from then on he resolved to approach his days differently. He learned to say thank you for things that happened to him, and to quickly let go of negative thoughts that came to mind. Though it's difficult to change a lifetime habit, and there were many bad days along with the good, Braden made tremendous improvement by truly becoming grateful for and learning from his hurdles.

In order to heal, it often becomes necessary to change how we see things. In order to change how we see things, we sometimes need to change our beliefs. In order to change our beliefs, we might need a new perspective, or some new insight. That doesn't happen easily as our typical reaction is to defend our beliefs, not change them. We are looking for an answer that fits inside the framework of beliefs we already have. As Braden discovered, we can get stuck in a rut of sickness or depression with no apparent way out.

When we feel peace, we feel safe, and healing and wellness naturally occur. Choosing faith over fear allows us to feel the peace of the Safe Box and enjoy the blessings of health.

Let's summarize what we have learned in this chapter.

1. **Law #2 of Healing and Wellness states – Correct Emotional Choices lead to healing and wellness.**
2. **Emotional survival is just as important as physical survival.**
3. **In the vivid memory are emotions to be dealt with and lessons to be learned.**
4. **Say - *"I'm grateful God protected me and guided me through this."***
5. **We must correctly identify the CAUSE of our problems.**
6. **Forgiveness of self and others allows healing to occur.**
7. **We are grateful for the experience because of the lessons it teaches us.**

THE EMOTIONAL ADD TWO PLAN

One way to feel this change within, and let go of current stress and past memories, is the *Emotional Add Two Plan.*

Take two negative situations, experiences, or memories out of your Unsafe Box and add them to your Safe Box. Work on those for a day, being grateful they are as good as they are, and grateful they weren't any worse. If you believe in God, be thankful for his help in dealing with them. The next day add two more stressful situations or experiences to your Safe Box, and work on those for a day. Continue to Add Two stresses or memories to your Safe Box each day, until you feel your Unsafe Box is empty.

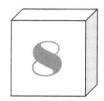

THE NUTRITIONAL SAFE BOX

Shortly after arriving in chiropractic college in 1979, my wife, Debi, broke out in a rash. We took her into the clinic at the college to see if we could get some help. Several interns looked at her and gave a variety of opinions as to what they thought caused the rash. Dr. Ted Morter happened to be visiting the school that day, and someone invited him into the room to get his opinion. Dr. Morter looked at Debi and said, *"You have a toxic liver. Eat three grapefruit a day for three days, and you will be fine."*

We were a little startled at such a "diagnosis". Toxic liver, what's that? What does a liver have to do with a skin rash? What do you mean by toxic? We didn't understand what Dr. Morter was talking about, but we did understand *"eat three grapefruit a day for three days"*, so that is what Debi did. In three days her rash was gone.

TREATING THE CAUSE

That was our introduction to nutrition, and to the concept that food has a significant impact on the health of our bodies. What we eat does make a difference! The study of nutrition and its application to health has been a major part of my life ever since. Poor nutrition is a major cause of the symptoms a person has, second only to emotions. By "nutrition" I mean anything we put into our body by eating, drinking, breathing, rubbing onto the skin, and so on. By "emotions" I mean anything having to do with the mind – meaning thoughts, feelings, and memories.

So far in this book we have talked about interfering with the body automatic as a way of producing health problems. We have seen how negative thoughts and feelings do this. In Chapter 6, we talked about the *4 Laws of Healing and Wellness*. The third law we listed there was **Correct Nutritional Choices Lead to Healing and Wellness.** In this chapter we will talk about what the proper nutritional choices are which will allow us to be in the **Nutritional Safe Box**.

It is important to remember that with any symptom or condition we have, we need to get to the cause. Trying to eat your way out of an emotional problem, or exercise your way out of a nutritional problem, or think your way out of a physical problem is not very effective. Though doing better in any of those areas may help, the results will be less than desirable when we don't treat the cause. We always have to get to the source of the problem for true healing to take place.

Many, many books have been written on the subject of nutrition. If a person were to study them all, he would come away totally confused. There is research that backs almost every diet you can imagine. But that is not the only confusing thing. You only have to go to another part of the world and try some of their food to question some of our dietetic ideas. What we consider a staple and necessary part of our diets may not even exist in theirs. It becomes very difficult to say specific foods are necessary when they may not even be available.

I recently attended a two day seminar on nutrition that I expected would extol the virtues of fruits and vegetables. I was shocked when study after study was projected on the screen showing the importance of consuming large amounts of protein. According to the presenter, one should be eating meat three times a day. I strongly disagree with this school of thought. Yet the seminar was good for me in that I was reminded again of the many varying opinions there are on what good nutrition is.

So how do we know what to believe when it comes to nutrition?

EATING IN THE NUTRITIONAL SAFE BOX

Bruce, a good friend of mine who was thirty years old, decided to take up running again. He had been somewhat of a runner before but it had been two years since he had pounded the pavement. In that time he had also changed his life style, giving up soda pop, cutting way back on sweets and eating significantly more fruits, vegetables and whole grains. He decided not to push himself as he began running, but just take it easy. He thought a fifteen minute run would be plenty. After fifteen minutes, he still felt very fresh and decided to run further. Bruce continued to run and run, amazed at how good he felt. After six miles he finally stopped, not that he felt he needed to, but that he was concerned about how he would feel the next day. To his surprise, he woke up feeling fine with hardly any stiffness or soreness at all. The difference in what he expected, he attributed to his new life style.

What changes had Bruce made in his way of living?

Bruce had greatly decreased the amount of refined and processed food he was eating and significantly increased his consumption of fruits, vegetables and whole grains. He was giving his body much better quality "fuel" and his body was responding very favorably to the change.

ALKALINE ASH AND ACID ASH FOODS

There is an important concept we need to explain here that is really an essential key to health and diet. When food is digested in the body, an ash is produced. This residue is very similar in concept to the ash that remains after wood is burned. This ash is of three types - acid, alkaline, or neutral. Our body itself is alkaline and to keep it that way we need to consume mostly alkaline ash foods, which are foods high in alkaline minerals. If we consume too many acid ash foods, our body will then become too acid. If the cells of the body become too acid they will not be able to function, or function poorly and eventually disease will result.

The affect of alkaline and acid ash foods on the body is a powerful yet overlooked principle that has been known for over one hundred years. Henry C. Sherman wrote about it in 1915. He said,

"The presence of potassium carbonate (potash) in wood ashes is familiar to everyone and accounts for the fact that wood ashes are alkaline or basic. Similarly those parts of plants which are used for food in the form of fruits and vegetables yield, on burning, a basic or alkaline ash...capable of neutralizing acids such as the sulfuric acid produced in the protein metabolism...Thus the predominance of base-forming elements among the ash constituents of fruits and vegetables is of great value to the body in facilitating the maintenance of the normal neutrality of the blood and tissues." (Henry C. Sherman, *Food Products,* 1915, p. 352)

Here is a list of some common alkaline ash and acid ash foods.

Common Alkaline Ash Foods			Common Acid Ash Foods		
Almonds	Dates	Parsnips	Bacon	Eggs	Pork
Apples	Figs, Dried	Peaches	Barley	Flour,	Prunes
Apricots	Grapefruit	Pears	grain	white	Rice
Avocados	Grapes	Pineapple	Beef	Flour,	Salmon
Bananas	Green beans	Potatoes,	Blueberries	wheat	Sardines
Barley juice	Green peas	sweet	Bran,	Fish	Sausage
Beans, dried	Lemons	Potatoes,	wheat	Honey	Scallops
Beet greens	Lettuce	white	Bran, oat	Lamb	Shrimp
Beets	Lima beans	Radishes	Bread,	Lentils	Spaghetti
Blackberries	dry	Raisins	white	Lobster	Squash,
Broccoli	Lima beans	Raspberries	Bread,	Milk,	winter
Brussel	green	Rutabagas	wheat	pasteurized	Sunflower
Sprouts	Limes	Sauerkraut	Butter	Macaroni	seeds
Cabbage	Milk, raw	Soy beans	Carob	Oatmeal	Turkey
Carrots	Millet	Spinach	Cheese	Oysters	Veal
Cauliflower	Molasses	Strawberries	Chicken	Peanut	Walnuts
Celery	Mushrooms	Tangerines	Cod	Butter	Wheat
Chard	Muskmelons	Tomatoes	Corn	Peanuts	germ
Cucumbers	Onions	Watermelon	Crackers	Plums	Yogurt

(Chart adapted from Dr. M. Ted Morter Jr., *An Apple a Day,* BEST Research Inc., 1996, 51-52)

As you can see from the chart, fruits and vegetables are the major alkaline ash foods. Even fruits that are acidic, like lemons, oranges and grapefruit leave an alkaline ash when digested.

Meats, grains, and dairy products are the major acid ash foods. Neutral ash foods are mostly oils and refined sugars. Their ash is neutral but they do have an acidifying effect on the body as they are burned for fuel.

Authors and researchers who understand the ash concept suggest that the ideal diet to keep the body alkaline and healthy would be about "seventy-five percent fruits and vegetables, and twenty-five percent high-protein meat, dairy and grain products" (Dr. M. Ted Morter Jr, *Fell's Know it All Guide to Health and Wellness,* Frederick Fell, Dec 2000, 57). Said another way, about three out of four bites of food should be from the alkaline ash side of the chart. That will vary from day to day and from season to season, but on the average seventy-five percent is a good goal, and will keep us in the Nutritional Safe Box.

Though meat and dairy are allowed in the twenty-five percent of acid ash foods, they are not necessary. There are many who are vegetarian or vegan, who can testify to this. One well known author on this subject is John A. McDougall, M.D. He advocates a whole food starch-centered diet, one high in wheat, rice, potatoes and beans. He has written numerous books and articles on how starches have been the main food source since the beginning of mankind, and of starches' health benefits. His website www.drmcdougall.com has a tremendous amount of excellent information on the virtues of plant foods, as well as many wonderful recipes.

Even the lowly, and much maligned potato is a wonderful health food when consumed in its entirety. One of my patients, Tina finally got serious about losing weight, and lost one hundred pounds in six months. How did she do it? Every day she ate lots of green beans and five baked potatoes. She cut out all white flour and white sugar and she walked five miles a day. That's not the most exciting diet, but she felt great, had lots of energy, wasn't hungry, and reached her goal.

THE NUTRITIONAL UNSAFE BOX – TOO MUCH ACID

Question: *What is in meats, grains, and dairy products that cause the acid ash?*

The acid ash results from protein breakdown. Protein leaves strong acid residues such as nitric acid, sulfuric acid, phosphoric acid and uric acid when digested. One cause of gout, for example, is too much uric acid resulting from eating too much protein. These acids must be neutralized by alkaline minerals such as sodium, potassium, and calcium and then eliminated by the kidneys. There are not enough minerals in these foods to neutralize the acid, so the minerals must be pulled from the body's reserves. Too much protein can lead to a loss of important minerals resulting in osteoporosis, kidney stones, muscle cramps and numerous other conditions.

The March 2009 *Readers Digest* published an article entitled, "A New Way to Keep Bones Strong", in which it shared new research from Tufts University. The article said that too much meat and grain in the diet makes the body acid and leaches calcium out of the bones, leading to osteoporosis. It stated, *"In contrast, fruits and vegetables create a skeleton-friendly alkaline environment."* A recommended solution was to *"Include at least two vegetables or fruit servings at every meal."* (A New Way to Keep Bones Strong, *Readers Digest,* March 2009, p 83)

Though this research may be new to some, I learned it thirty years ago, and as mentioned earlier, it wasn't new then. The alkaline ash and acid ash concept goes back to at least 1907 when a paper entitled "The Balance of Acid Forming and Base Forming Element in Food" by HC Shelton was published in the *Journal of Biological Chemistry.* It is good to see modern researchers verifying such "ancient" information, and getting it into main stream media.

Question: *How much protein should we consume then?*

Let's figure it this way. The main purpose protein serves in our diet is for growth and repair. A baby doubles his birth weight in about six months on a diet consisting of only mother's milk. At no point in his life will he ever grow that fast again. Since the perfect food for a baby is his mother's milk, and the first six months of his life is his greatest need for protein, there must be a lot of protein in mothers' milk, right?

Wrong. Mother's milk is only 1 to 1.5 percent protein. Since we will never grow again so rapidly, we can assume that there would never be a time in our lives when our diets would need to be more than 1.5 percent protein.

The following chart shows that the amount of protein in the milk of an animal varies depending upon the rate of growth of the young of that species.

COMPARISON OF THE MILKS OF DIFFERENT SPECIES		
	Per cent Protein	Days to double birth weight
Human	1.2	180
Mare	2.4	60
Cow	3.3	47
Goat	4.1	19
Dog	7.1	8
Cat	9.5	7
Rat	11.8	4.5

(Source: John A. McDougall, MD, *The McDougall Plan,* 101)

A baby rat needs a higher protein amount because it doubles its birth weight in 4.5 days. A human baby takes much longer and needs only 1.2% protein.

At the turn of the century, recommended protein intake was more than one hundred grams (about four ounces) a day. It is now estimated that an adult human can do very well on as little as twenty grams (two-thirds of an ounce). The discrepancy is due to how recommended daily allowances were established. Studies to determine the needs of humans were not done on people but on rats. They were then extrapolated to quantities for humans. The fallacy of this can be seen when we compare the milk of a mother rat to that of a mother human. The protein content of rat's milk is almost twelve percent, considerably more than that of human milk at one and one-half percent. Twelve percent is a logical percentage though when we consider that a new born rat takes only four days to double its birth weight as well as a very short time to mature. (See John A. McDougall, MD, *The McDougall Plan,* 95)

The World Health Organization recommends that the average working man, who eats three thousand calories a day, should consume thirty-seven grams of protein. The average woman consuming two thousand three hundred calories a day would need twenty-nine grams. If a person simply ate three thousand calories of white potatoes in a day, he would have consumed eighty grams of highly usable protein. Once again we can see that it is almost impossible to be protein deficient. (See John A. McDougall, MD, *The McDougall Plan,* 95)

Some may question whether they will get enough of the essential amino acids when they decrease their consumption of animal products. Essential amino acids are the building blocks of protein. They need to be consumed in food as the body doesn't produce them. As the amino acids are consumed, the body uses them to "build" the protein specific to the area of the body where it is needed. The initial recommended daily allowance of amino acids was also based on studies with rats and thus are exaggerated. When compared with mother's milk, we again see that a combination of fruits and vegetables gives us more than enough protein.

Question: *What are some foods besides mother's milk that consist of one and one half percent protein?*

Let's look at a list of the protein content of some common foods on the chart on the next page. Only some fruits fall short of 1.5 percent protein as well as watery type vegetables such as cucumbers.

You will notice that one would have to be a total fruitarian to be in danger of not having enough protein – yet remember that 1.5% is the most we would ever need.

PROTEIN CONTENT (PER 100 GRAMS)

Fruit Protein	%	Vegetables Protein	%	Other Plants	%	Animal Protein	%
Apples	0.4	Beans	2.4	Oatmeal	14.2	Milk	3.5
Bananas	1.2	Broccoli	3.3	Wheat	13.8	Cheeses	20-25
Grapes	1.3	Carrots	1.2	Rice	9.0	Eggs	12.8
Oranges	0.9	Cucumbers	0.7	Corn	11.4	Poultry	22-28
Peaches	0.7	Potatoes	2.0	Beans	20-30	Beef	15-20
Pears	0.6	Spinach	2.3	Almonds	18.6	Fish	15-20
Raspberries	1.7	Tomatoes	1.0	Pecans	9.4	Pork	15-18

(Chart adapted from Dr. Ted Morter Jr., *An Apple a Day,* BEST Research Inc., 1996, 229-236)

It's easy to see that it is almost impossible to **not** get enough protein in our diet. It's also easy to see how simple it is to get too much protein in our diets. Because of the highly acid residue that is left over when protein is digested, our body can eventually become toxic. Excess protein must be considered as one of the main causes of disease in our modern society today, and a major contributor to the Nutritional Unsafe Box.

Question: *Would it be better then to eat poultry or fish than red meat?*

Our society has become very much aware of the adverse effects of too much fat in the diet, so many have suggested leaner cuts of meat, poultry, or fish as an alternative to the "traditional" roast, steak, or hamburger. If one does this he will definitely consume less fat. But, if he eats the same size portion, he simply consumes more protein, in place of the fat. For example, regular hamburger would be about sixteen percent protein, while most fish would be about eighteen percent, chicken about twenty-one percent, and turkey about twenty-four percent. We simply trade one problem for another when we substitute protein for fat. The better solution is to eat more alkaline ash foods.

Question: *What about milk?*

Many of us have grown up being told milk is necessary to good health. But is it really? Because it's such a big part of our culture, we don't realize that most people in the world have diets that contain no dairy products at all. That should make us wonder. Dairy products are one of the leading causes of food allergies, which should also tell us something.

Most people's concern in limiting milk in their diet is that they will not be getting enough calcium. Calcium is one of the most plentiful of all minerals. It's found in virtually every food. Like protein, it's almost impossible to not consume enough calcium.

The major reason we see a deficiency of calcium in a person is not due to lack of consumption but due to too much protein and other acidifying foods. The Tufts University study quoted by the *Reader's Digest* mentioned above says too much meat and grain in the diet makes the body acid and leaches calcium out of the bone. Research has shown that when more than forty-seven grams of protein are consumed the body loses calcium in an effort to handle the acid ash. Since the average American diet contains more than forty-seven grams of protein, the average American eventually becomes deficient in calcium. That is one of the reasons we see so much osteoporosis and other nutritionally related diseases in our country today. (See M. Ted Morter, DC, *An Apple A Day,* BEST Research Inc, 1996, p 65)

A study on hip fractures due to osteoporosis compared the protein and calcium intake of people in ten different countries. The United States had the highest incidence of hip fractures per capita, with about 100 per 100,000 people. Americans also consumed the most protein and consumed the most calcium, mostly in the form of dairy products. The lower end of the study was Singapore and Hong Kong, with about 30 hip fractures per 100,000 people. Their population consumed the least amount of protein, calcium and dairy products. (See M. Ted Morter, DC, *An Apple A Day,* BEST Research Inc, 1996, p 66)

Part of the reason milk may not be the health food we think it should be is due to how it is processed. Between 1932 and 1942, Francis M. Pottenger M.D. studied 900 cats to determine the effects processed milk had on their bodies. This feeding experiment involved four groups of cats. One group received a diet of 2/3 raw milk, 1/3 raw meat and cod liver oil. The other groups received a diet of processed milk (either 2/3 pasteurized milk, 2/3 evaporated milk, or 2/3 sweetened condensed milk), plus 1/3 raw meat and cod liver oil. The more processed the milk, the worse the effect on the cats' health. The most marked deficiencies occurred in the cats eating the most processed food – the sweetened, condensed milk. The results of this now famous study are shown below.

POTTENGER CAT EXPERIMENT SUMMARY

FOOD	Raw Milk	Pasteurized Milk	Evaporated Milk	Condensed Milk
1st Generation	Remained healthy	Developed diseases and illnesses near end of life		
2nd Generation	Remained healthy	Developed diseases and illnesses in middle of life		
3rd Generation	Remained healthy	Developed diseases and illnesses in beginning of life; many died before six months of age;		
4th Generation	Remained healthy	No fourth generation was produced: either third generation parents were sterile, or fourth generation cats were aborted before birth		

(Francis M. Pottenger, M.D., *Pottenger's Cats, A Study in Nutrition,* Price-Pottenger Nutrition Foundation, 15)

Though humans are not cats, there is a lesson to be learned from this study. The more processed a food is, the more deficient in nutrients it becomes. That will undoubtedly have a profound effect upon our health, and the health of our future generations.

In my experience milk is definitely not the health food it has been promoted to be. Cutting back on dairy products or eliminating them all together has helped many of my patients with chronic ailments such as sinus congestion, allergies, asthma, rashes, bed wetting, ear infections and joint pains. Milk products can be tolerated by some, and if consumed, should be in the twenty-five per cent of acid ash food we mentioned above.

Raw milk is an alkaline ash food so is not acidifying to the body like homogenized and pasteurized milk. But it hard to come by and not necessary. Therefore milk products are nice for an occasional treat, not as a major part of one's diet. Fruits and vegetables are the most valuable alkalizing health foods.

Question: *The previous chart indicates that grains are about fourteen percent protein. Is that too much protein?*

As with meat and dairy, it depends on how much grain you consume. For example, I treated a person with back problems who was a non-meat eater. He only improved about fifty percent and then no further. I finally asked him what his diet was like. He said that basically all he was eating was grains and some dried beans. That was too much protein and so I had him go on fruits and vegetables for five days. By the third day his body was no longer so acidic, his back was fine, and we didn't need to treat him any further.

Wheat, like milk, is one of the major causes of food allergies. Many people also have a difficult time digesting grains high in gluten. There are three things a person can do that will help the body to better handle wheat and other grains.

1. **Don't consume too much grain.** – Grain is an acid ash food. It should be in the twenty-five percent category. Adding more fruits and vegetables to the diet will often help, like it did with the patient above.

2. **Eat whole grains, not refined grains.** – Whole grain products don't cause nearly as many problems as refined grain products. White flour is deficient in most minerals and vitamins, and doesn't have much fiber. Many studies have been done, similar to Pottenger's studies, demonstrating the unhealthy effects of refined grains. (See John A. McDougall, MD, *The McDougall Plan,* 114-127)

3. **Use sprouted grains.** – Sprouting causes a little miracle to take place. Enzymes which have lain dormant are activated. They begin to break down the

complex starch molecules into simple sugars, they convert saturated fats into free fatty acids, and they split long chain proteins into free amino acids. This makes the grain much easier for our bodies to handle, and we don't have the allergic reactions. In addition, vitamin and mineral content is increased up to a thousand times. Also the sprouted grain produces an alkaline rather than an acid ash when digested, and thus will add to the alkalinity of our body rather than take away from it, as the unsprouted grain does.

WEIGHT LOSS

With two thirds of North Americans being over weight, weight loss is an important subject to address.

The basic energy source for our bodies is glucose, a simple sugar. We burn it as fuel to give us energy. Glucose is a major component of carbohydrates and carbohydrates are a major component of starch. All plant foods contain starch. Animal foods do not. A person eating a large amount of fruits, vegetables and grains would consume a large amount of starchy foods. Dr. John McDougall says this is the way it should be. He says, *"The basic metabolism of the body is genetically encoded to run most efficiently on starches"* (McDougall Newsletter, March 2009, Vol. 8, No. 3, p.2).

What are starches? The Colombia Encyclopedia defines starches this way. *"In green plants starch is produced by photosynthesis; it is one of the chief forms in which plants store food. It is stored most abundantly in tubers (e.g., the white potato), roots (e.g., the sweet potato), seeds, and fruits; it appears in the form of grains that differ in size, shape, and markings."* (http://encyclopedia2.thefreedictionary.com/starch)

Though we are saying starch is an excellent food source, you may have heard statements like, *"Don't eat starches, because rice and potatoes turn to sugar, which turns to fat, making you gain weight"*. This just isn't true. Just looking at different world populations affirms this. Those living in Japan, China, Korea, Thailand, Indonesia, and the Philippines eat mostly rice and vegetables, and are not overweight. In rural Mexico they eat corn, beans, and squash and are not overweight.

In Peru, potatoes are a staple, and in New Guinea sweet potatoes. Again, the native populations are not overweight. *"Worldwide, populations with the highest consumption of starch are the trimmest and fittest... They also have extremely low rates of diabetes, arthritis, gallbladder disease, constipation, indigestion, multiple sclerosis, heart disease, and cancers of the breast, prostate, and colon."* (McDougall Newsletter, March 2009, Vol. 8, No. 3, p.2) Take these same people and put them on the typical Western diet, and they will eventually be overweight and unhealthy as well.

Why is this so? Dr. McDougall offers this explanation, *"Starches, like corn, beans, potatoes, and rice, are abundant in* **carbohydrates,** *dietary fiber, and are very low in fat. Appetite satisfaction begins with physically filling the stomach. Compared to cheese (4 calories per gram), meat (4 calories per gram), and oils (9 calories per gram),* **starches, at only one calorie per gram,** *are very calorie dilute. In the simplest terms, starches physically will fill you up with a fraction—one-fourth— of the calories as will cheese, meat, and oil. Furthermore ...eating carbohydrates leads to long-term satiety, enduring for hours between meals; whereas the fats in a meal have little impact on satiety—people are left wanting more food when they eat fats and oils."* (McDougall Newsletter, March 2009, Vol. 8, No. 3, p.3)

A four nation study by Linda van Horn of Northwestern University concluded, *"Without exception, the thinnest people on Earth eat the most carbohydrates. The people who eat the most protein are actually the heaviest."* (As reported by CNN on March 6, 2004 http://www.mickormackiga.com/files/CNN_com)

Generally, a cup of grains or beans contains about 200 calories and a cup of fruits or vegetables about 100 calories. A weight loss program permitting 1300 calories a day would allow about 13 cups of fruits and vegetables, or 6 cups of grains and beans, or some combination of that – plenty of food to give you energy and satisfy your appetite. Contrast that with the typical fast food meal of a hamburger, shake, and fries, which contains 1300 calories, not at all close to being enough food for the typical person on an average day.

Or try eating twice that amount, 2600 calories a day. You

can see it would be easy to double the hamburger, shake and fries, but try 26 cups of fruits and vegetables or 12 cups of grains and beans a day. You would be full long before you could reach that amount. It's easy to see why people in native cultures don't worry about weight loss.

THE SPILLOVER PRINCIPLE

When my wife, Debi, had a rash and Dr. Morter told her it was from a toxic liver and to eat three grapefruit a day for three days, it opened a whole new world of learning for us. I have enjoyed studying and teaching about nutrition and toxicity a great deal since.

There are many things that affect our level of toxicity. One way of becoming too toxic is by becoming too acidic. We can do this by eating too much acid ash food as we have discussed. Too much acid ash food can overwhelm the body. Some acid ash food is okay, but overall our diets should consist of 75 percent alkaline ash foods.

Too much soda pop, tea and coffee will also increase that toxic load as they are also acid. The acid has to be neutralized, and the liver has a significant role in that. The liver is the major organ for cleansing. If the liver can't keep up with the filtering out of toxins, then back-up systems will have to help out, and symptoms will begin to develop. Like trying to fill a bucket too full, you get a spillover. A skin rash is a common spillover symptom. So are a runny nose and an upset stomach.

Another source of toxicity is the huge amount of chemicals in our foods and environment. *A Consumer's Dictionary of Food Additives* is a five hundred page book listing twelve thousand different chemicals added to our foods mostly for enhanced looks, taste, and preservation. What kind of impact do these chemicals have on our body, individually and collectively? A single slice of bread may have *"sixteen chemicals in it to keep it feeling fresh"* (Ruth Winter, M.S., *A Consumer's Dictionary of Food Additives"*, Three Rivers Press, 32). Multiply those sixteen chemicals by all the other chemicals we ingest or are exposed to in a day, and you can see what a huge undertaking it is to keep our body clean.

The major reason we do so well is the marvelous organ

we have called a liver. It performs about five hundred functions that we know of, detoxification being one of the most important. It deals with nutrients, drugs and other toxins absorbed into the blood stream via the intestines, skin and lungs. *"It is a remarkably resilient organ and the human body can withstand the loss of up to two thirds of the normal liver without the development of liver insufficiency."* (http://www.liver.co.uk/) But eventually it can get overwhelmed, and thankfully there are back up systems to compensate, or we would not survive. Though we may have symptoms we don't like, at least we are alive.

Here are three more ways to tell if your body is becoming too toxic, and your "bucket" is beginning to spill over.

1. **Stiff and Sore in the Morning** – If you are stiff and sore when you get up, and then loosen up as the day progresses, you are likely too toxic. The acid or toxins settle in your joints and muscles when you sleep, and you work them out as you move around.

2. **A headache behind your eyes** – If you frequently have a headache in your forehead behind your eyes, you typically are too toxic. It will often be worse after eating, indicating that what you ate was not ideal for you.

3. **Smelling ammonia in the urine** – The smell of ammonia in your urine is also a toxic indicator. Excess protein leads to excess acid in the urine. If the urine gets too acid, damage to the kidneys could occur. The body, in its wisdom, will make ammonia, an alkaline by-product that protects the kidneys. Smelling ammonia indicates a person has become overly acid.

EMPTY FOODS

Another nutritional reason for symptoms is a deficiency of essential nutrients like vitamins, minerals, amino acids, fatty acids, enzymes, antioxidants, phytonutrients, and water. If we are deficient in these, then our body doesn't have enough of the right building blocks to be healthy. One reason our bodies become deficient in these nutrients is food processing or food refining.

We should eat our food as close to the way God created it as possible. When food is processed it loses a great deal of its nutritional value. In general, the more food we eat in its natural state and the less it is refined without additives, the healthier it will be for us.

Pottenger's study with cats demonstrated this effect way back in the 1940's. Cooking food destroys some of its nutrients. Refining food through chemical or mechanical means removes even more. Which of the following foods, Food A or Food B, would you choose to eat if you were thinking of your health?

Vitamins	Food A	Food B	Minerals	Food A	Food B
B1	0.14 mg	0 mg	Potassium	450 mg	0 mg
B2	0.14 mg	0 mg	Phosphorus	50 mg	0 mg
B3	0.20 mg	0 mg	Calcium	100 mg	0 mg
B5	1.20 mg	0 mg	Magnesium	150 mg	0 mg
B6	0.40 mg	0 mg	Zinc	.10 mg	0 mg
C	4.30 mg	0 mg	Iron	8.0 mg	0 mg
D	27.0 IU	0 IU	Copper	.10 mg	0 mg
E	.004 IU	0 IU	Manganese	3.0 mg	0 mg

(Adapted from International Starch Institute
http://home3.inet.tele.dk/starch/isi/starch/sugar.htm)

Food B is white table sugar, which is stripped of all vitamins, minerals, fiber, amino acids and trace elements during the refining process. Food A is the sugar cane from which the sugar is made. The essential vitamins and minerals are destroyed or separated out during processing. Consuming Food B and expecting our body to make something beneficial out of it is like asking a carpenter to build a house without any materials.

Refining wheat berries to white flour also creates an empty or near-empty food. Fifty to ninety percent of the essential vitamins, minerals and other nutrients are lost in that process. The body is amazing in its ability to adapt to the things we do to it, but it eventually catches up to us. We can't run on bad fuel forever.

Though researchers do not all agree on what a good diet is, I have never heard one suggest we need to consume more refined and processed foods. There is a universal consensus that refined, "empty" foods are detrimental to our health.

Blair was thirty-one years old and said he felt like he was ninety. He had not been able to work for two weeks. His wife helped him into our office as he was not able to walk on his own. He was experiencing fatigue, memory loss, slurred speech, and had a difficult time putting a sentence together. He had pain in all his joints, burning in his arms and numbness in his hands. He had migraine headaches for twelve years and joint pain for nine. Eight months earlier is when the forgetfulness began. For the past three months he had been having episodes where he would "blank out" and become unresponsive. A week earlier he had passed out and was taken to the emergency room. An MRI and other tests ruled out a brain tumor.

Blair's symptoms indicated to me that he was very acidic, so I asked him about his diet. He said his typical menu was cereal for breakfast, processed meat and white bread sandwiches for lunch, and a steak and baked potato for supper. He didn't eat any other vegetables and maybe had one piece of fruit a week. He drank several cups of coffee a day, though not the thirty-six a day he used to drink in college, and drank very little water.

I explained to Blair how deficiencies in nutrients and being overly acidic could create the symptoms he was having. I had him add two pieces of fruit and two vegetables a day to his diet, take a good nutritional supplement, and drink plenty of water. Within a week he was no longer blanking out and experiencing memory loss. He was able to return to work for four hours a day. Within two weeks Blair was back to work full time, had much more energy, and no more pain, numbness or burning. Within a month he felt like he was thirty-one years old again.

ROBBING FROM PETER TO PAY PAUL

According to the Spillover Principle, if our body gets too toxic for our liver to handle, there is a spillover into some other part of the body to compensate. There is another equally important action our body will take if a deficiency becomes too great. That is called "Robbing from Peter to Pay Paul".

*David came into my office with a hives on his forearms.
They had popped up a week earlier and were driving him crazy.
In addition, he had been having quite a few more leg cramps the
last couple of months, which were helped by taking potassium.*

The hives were a good hint that David was eating too much acid ash food and getting a spillover, so I asked him about it. He had been laid off work two months earlier, and had started drinking a mug or more of soda pop a day as he sat around the house. In addition to that, a candy bar had become a daily treat. Also, "in order to get healthy", he had started eating a bowl of cracked wheat cereal every morning.

If the diet is too acid, as David's was, alkaline minerals like potassium are used to neutralize that excess acid. If David's diet is also deficient in potassium, where is he going to get enough potassium to take care of the acid? The body has a good reservoir of potassium in the muscles so it robs potassium from the muscles in his legs (Peter) to give to the liver and other organs (Paul) to get rid of the excess acid. He now suffers with leg cramps due to a deficiency of potassium. It's a good emergency system, but not one David wants to have very long. He can take a supplement which relieves the cramps, but he is now treating the symptom and not the cause. Eventually other symptoms may occur. In David's case, it was hives.

David quit the pop and the candy bar and even the cracked wheat cereal. He started to drink lots of water and eat more fruits and vegetables. Within a week the itching was gone, and only a little redness on his forearms remained. Once he became more alkaline and less acid, he then could start eating the cereal again without consequences. The cracked wheat is acidic, but when balanced with enough alkaline foods, is very good for him. The pop and candy bar have no nutritional value and only detract from his health.

Another good example of how the body will rob nutrients from one part to fill the need of another is osteoporosis. *Alice was eighty years old, and bent over as a result of weak and calcium deficient bones.*

Though her bones were deficient in calcium, a blood test showed normal levels of blood calcium. How can the body be so deficient in calcium in one place, and perfectly normal in the other? Our blood is our life line and it is vital to our survival that our blood calcium level stays normal. Alice's bones were a good reservoir to draw from in time of need, so her body robbed from Peter, her bones, to pay Paul, her blood. Alice understood the concept we just explained, changed her diet dramatically and her bone density increased twenty-five percent in twelve months.

SLOW GOING

There is one caution I should add as you think about improving your diet. Never change your eating habits too rapidly. Your body is used to what you have been putting into it. If you alter what your body is accustomed to, too quickly, it may make you feel sick. Toxins are stored in your body, and are released when you eat better. This "cleansing" can cause spillover symptoms if it occurs too fast. Headaches, stiffness and soreness, sinus drainage, skin rashes, nausea and other symptoms may occur. So go slow. Take your time as you improve your diet. Your main objective is to gradually increase the amount of alkaline ash foods until they are 75 percent of what you consume.

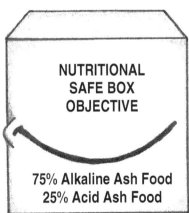

NUTRITIONAL SAFE BOX OBJECTIVE

75% Alkaline Ash Food
25% Acid Ash Food

THE NUTRITIONAL ADD TWO PLAN

The program we recommend to move from the Nutritional Unsafe Box to the Nutritional Safe Box is the *Add Two Plan.*

Add 2 fruits, 2 vegetables and 2 glasses of water to your

daily diet for a week, in addition to those you already consume. If you handle that well, without any symptoms, then add 2 more servings of each for another week. If cleansing symptoms do develop, cut back on the fruit. Keep adding 2 more fruits, vegetables and glasses of water a week until you are eating 75% alkaline ash foods and water is 75% of your liquid intake.

Darwin had implemented the Add Two Plan. He had gradually added fruits and vegetables until they were a big part of his daily diet. He said, *"I know the program works. I went skiing two weeks ago, and skied really hard the first day, as I always do. For the past twenty years, since I was fifteen, I have done that and have always been extremely stiff and sore the second day. This time I ate lots of fruit and drank lots of water after skiing that first day. I didn't drink any alcohol or eat any junk. The second day I was hardly stiff at all. I couldn't believe how good I felt! I skied just as I did the first day. Eating this way really makes a difference."*

Darwin had learned a good and valuable lesson about the importance of eating alkaline ash foods. But he wasn't done learning. He had a blood test done and found that his cholesterol numbers were all high, his total cholesterol being about 260. Darwin wasn't surprised at this as he still ate a lot of animal protein. He especially loved to eat a big breakfast of bacon, eggs and sausage. We gave him a simple, general menu to follow which helped him greatly in making further changes to his diet and bringing down his cholesterol numbers.

THE IDEAL MENU

Here is the basic ideal menu we recommend you strive for as you implement the *Add Two Program*, and increase alkaline ash foods to 75%. (Adapted from M. Ted Morter, D.C., *The Nutrition Seminar,* BEST Research Inc., 1991, p 31)

> **Breakfast – Eat a fruit meal.**
> **Lunch – Eat a starch meal.**
> **Dinner – Eat a starch and protein meal.**

Eating fruit for breakfast is ideal. Fruit is quickly digested giving you energy within thirty minutes and enabling you to be mentally alert, physically active, and ready to begin your day. You could eat citrus fruits, bananas, mangos, grapes, smoothies, or whatever fruit you like. This meal is extremely alkalizing to your body. Your body spends your sleeping hours rejuvenating, healing and cleansing. It can continue this work in the morning if you don't load it down with a heavy meal. Most people are not very hungry in the morning and eating a grapefruit or orange or apple or couple of bananas is very satisfying. If you are used to a big breakfast, it may take a few weeks to get used to eating fruit as you begin the day. You can have a fruit or fruit smoothie or fresh juice several times during the morning if you wish. You will be amazed at how alert and energetic you will feel.

Starches are better eaten at noon. They generally take from one to two hours to digest and are more of a sustaining type of meal. Sample meals would be vegetable salads, soups containing lots of vegetables, and potatoes, beets, dried beans, brown rice, corn, and so on. Vegetable starches are generally alkalizing and grain starches generally acidifying, so you would want to consume mostly vegetables as you strive for 75 percent alkaline ash.

Protein meals are better eaten in the evening. Protein is necessary for building and repairing the body, and repair and regeneration is one of the purposes of sleep. So eating protein in the evening for dinner gives the body the essential building blocks it needs to rebuild while sleeping. Protein generally takes 3-4 hours to digest and is more efficiently done while you are resting in the evening than while working during the day. Meals should include lots of vegetables and possibly grain, nut or animal products. Again, vegetable starches are alkalizing and most grains, nuts and animal products acidifying, so emphasize the vegetables.

Snacks should mostly be fruit, and beverages should mainly be pure water and occasionally juice.

A HEALTH AND WEIGHT LOSS SECRET

Dale had digestive and cholesterol problems and wanted to lose eighty pounds.

When I suggested eating fruit for breakfast, Dale didn't think he could do it. He was a rancher and said his work load was just too much to survive on fruit. He needed his bacon, eggs and pancakes to give him the energy he needed. In fact, he said his big breakfasts were hardly enough as he was famished by noon.

I explained to Dale that the fruit would give him energy right away, and that his "famished" feeling was likely that of a full stomach becoming empty. Bacon, eggs and pancakes would digest in his stomach for three or four hours, and then empty into his small intestine. That emptying sensation he felt at 9:00 or 10:00 in the morning had been interpreted as "hunger". In reality, it was an emptying sensation. By eating fruit he wouldn't have that famished or hungry feeling since he wouldn't get that emptying sensation.

Dale reported back to me that on the first day he started the *Ideal Menu* he had two oranges for breakfast. He worked right through the noon hour without even thinking about food again. He couldn't believe that the oranges had sustained him that long, and was grateful for his new-found health and weight loss secrets. They were an important step in his being able to cut back on the amount of food he ate and achieving the health and weight loss goals he had. Here are three secrets David discovered by eating fruit for breakfast rather than bacon, eggs, and pancakes.

1. He had more energy.
2. He didn't get hungry.
3. He ate less food during the day.

By slowly building up to following the *Ideal Menu* outlined, and gradually cutting back on pop, tea, coffee, animal products and refined, processed foods you will have a cleaner and more efficient body. You will discover your own health and weight loss secrets as you choose to live in the Nutritional Safe Box.

JUICING FOR HEALTH

As you strive to improve your diet, a good natural nutritional supplement is very beneficial in helping your body rebuild and regain its health. One of the best is a glass of freshly made juice. Carrot juice and apple juice are my favorite, but any fruit or vegetable will do. Of course you need a juicer, and time to make the juice. It's time and money well spent. Fresh juice is a highly concentrated source of vitamins, minerals and other nutrients and is a delicious way to replace missing nutrients from empty foods you have consumed, and repay Peter who you robbed from to pay Paul.

Juice is especially good for you because it is so easy to digest, giving you an abundance of nutrients with very little effort on the part of your body. Energy your body would have used to digest solid food can be used to cleanse and repair instead. You will want to begin slowly if you are not used to eating lots of fruits and vegetables. A couple of ounces of juice a day may be plenty. Drink it as a snack or as a meal, but not with a lot of other food. The nutrients are so high, fresh juice is a meal by itself. You can gradually work up until you are drinking 10-16 ounces a day as a nutritional supplement. Drinking too much juice too fast may cause uncomfortable cleansing or "detoxing" symptoms. If that happens, cut back on the juice until the symptoms go away and then increase the juice again.

If you are not able to do fresh juice, there are many good natural supplements on the market. Of course there are many that are not so good, so you will want to do some research. The ones I like the best are concentrated from whole foods, are cold processed, and are ideally a liquid, like the IntraMax we sell in our office.

Let's review what it takes to live in the Nutritional Safe Box:

1. **The ideal diet is 75% alkaline ash foods, and 25% acid ash foods.**
2. **Too much acid ash food and too many nutrient deficient foods lead to toxicity.**
3. **Whole starches like brown rice, wheat, potatoes, and vegetables are very good for you and help you lose weight.**
4. **When the liver is overworked spillover symptoms occur.**

5. **The body will rob nutrients from "Peter" to pay a deficient "Paul", eventually leading to symptoms.**
6. **Go slow and *Add Two* fruits or vegetables as you improve your diet.**
7. **The *Ideal Menu* is fruit for breakfast, starches for lunch, and starches (mostly vegetables) and protein for dinner.**

We have highlighted some of the more important aspects of the Nutritional Safe Box in this chapter. If you would like more information on these nutritional concepts, go to our website www.3stepstohealyourself.com. Click on the *Help Yourself* section to watch free classes, videos and workshops and to download free articles and other information.

For more enlightenment on the scientific evidence supporting these nutritional concepts, you might consider reading the following books, or go to their authors' respective websites:

M. Ted Morter, D.C., *An Apple A Day,* BEST Research Inc., 1996 (www.morter.com)
Dr. John and Mary McDougall, *The McDougall Plan,* Ingram Book Co., 1983 (www.drmcdougall.com)
John A. McDougall, M.D., *The McDougall Plan for Maximum Weight Loss,* Penguin Books, Inc, 1994 (www.drmcdougall.com)
T. Colin Campbell, PhD, *The China Study,* BenBella Books, 2006 (www.tcollincampbell.org)
Joel Fuhrman, M.D., *Eat to Live,* Little, Brown and Company 2003 (www.drfuhrman.com)
Joel Fuhrman, M.C., *Eat for Health,* Gift of Health Press, 2008, (www.drfuhrman.com)
Steven G. Aldana, Ph.D., *The Culprit and The Cure,* Maple Mountain Press, 2005 (www.theculpritandthecure.com)
Russell L. Blaylock, M.D., *Excitotoxins, The Taste That Kills,* Health Press, 1997 (http://www.russellblaylockmd.com)

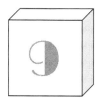

THE PHYSICAL SAFE BOX

Jerlyn came to see me with a stiff neck. She got better with a few treatments, but didn't improve as much as she should. That was a sign to me we were missing something. She then told me about her job. She was a secretary and spent half of the day with the telephone tucked between her ear and her shoulder taking orders and making notes. At the end of a work day, her neck was always worse. I asked about a head set, and she said that her boss had been intending to get one, but business was pretty tight, and they were just waiting for more money to come in. She had been doing this for six months, and it was apparent her neck wasn't going to get any better until she could change what she was physically doing to herself.

PHYSICAL REMINDERS

The fourth Law of Healing is **Correct Physical Choices lead to healing and wellness.**

Jerlyn was making an improper physical choice by how she held the phone, and it was keeping her from being well. Of these three causes, the emotional, nutritional and physical, the physical is typically, by far, the easiest one to figure out. We seem to naturally and quickly think, when a symptom arises, "*I wonder what I did?"* We rarely think, *"I wonder what I ate?* or *"I wonder what I thought?"*

As we spontaneously look to a physical cause of our symptoms, there is little need to expound on this concept, so this chapter is intentionally short. However, Jerlyn could use a few reminders and suggestions, and maybe you can too.

1. Be aware of posture and repetitive use type situations. Use proper tools, chairs and other equipment that take strain off your body.
2. Exercise is an essential component of good health and wellness. For the purpose of healing and staying well, a **brisk thirty minute walk five days a week** is adequate for most people. If you can't do that, then you need to gradually work up to that, or do some other comparable exercise. You should not exceed the speed that enables you to carry on a conversation.
3. A true physical injury can take two to three months to heal, so be patient. Ice is good for sprains and strains, heat for tense or tight muscles.
4. Six to eight hours of sleep a night is important to good health. If you don't sleep well, or are not rested when you wake up, there is likely an underlying emotional or nutritional cause.

AUTOMATIC HEALING

As we have said before, the body knows what to do. It never makes a mistake. When you are injured it will heal and repair the injury. There are two more important points to remember.

1. **If your body doesn't heal as expected, then there is another nutritional or emotional cause involved.**
2. **If you don't know what caused the symptom, then it is likely not physical, and you need to consider the nutritional and emotional.**

Let's consider the first. Rebecca had pain in her left side and back. She'd had a baby nine months earlier, and it had been there since. She said it felt like her rib cage had not come down after the delivery. She said, *"I wonder what I did?"* From what you have learned so far, might you have a suggestion as to why Rebecca was hurting?

Rebecca's body is not healing as expected, so there must be an emotional or nutritional cause. As it started with delivery, it would be wise to ask Rebecca how the delivery went. She said it was very difficult emotionally. She had labored for two weeks, but failed to progress, so she was induced. The cord was wrapped several times around her baby's neck, and they about lost her. This was her second child, so I asked about her first delivery. That one was more difficult physically than the second. She went through 38 hours of hard labor, and forceps were needed for delivery.

Could these memories be stored in Rebecca's Unsafe Box, contributing to her pain? Could the way Rebecca's second labor failed to progress be associated with the fear of another delivery similar to her first? We can use the analogy that holding onto these fearful memories was like she was holding out her arm for too long a period of time. When Rebecca understood the cause of her pain, she was able to figuratively "put her arm down". The muscles in her rib cage relaxed and she was pain free the rest of the day, the first time in nine months.

The next day her pain was back, though not as bad. Why? What had she done? She had simply "picked her arm back up", so to speak. She had once again picked up her fear. Rebecca realized that letting go of the physical experience of delivery was relatively easy, because it was over and in the past. Letting go of the fear of losing her baby, however, was not. That possibility still existed in the present and was something about which she thought frequently. Letting go of this fear required faith and a different perspective, and this was not easy.

Rebecca could not remain in a state of fear of losing her baby and remain pain free. Fear does not produce that type of outcome, only faith does. She needed to believe what she believes. By turning it over to God and trusting that his will would be done, which was her belief, she was able to, once again, let her rib cage relax. Once again she was able to experience immediate relief, but this was not an easy lesson and was one she would have to work on over and over again.

Now let's consider the second point mentioned above:

If you don't know what caused the symptom, then it is likely not physical, and again you need to consider the nutritional and emotional.

Suppose this happened to you. You are sitting at home with your daughter, having a fruit smoothie for breakfast. Your daughter is visiting with you about various things, and suddenly you feel your heart begin to race. You've had this happen many times before, and have been through medical tests that indicate your heart is fine. But here it goes again. Your blood pressure is high and heart rate is erratic. What do you do? What do you think?

If you are like April who came in with these symptoms, you think, *"I wonder what's wrong. I wonder what I did."*

You would have to conclude that your problem is not physical. You have already ruled that out with several medical tests, and you were just sitting and not exerting yourself. That leaves nutritional and emotional as the possible causes. All you had for breakfast was the fruit smoothie, with no caffeine or any other stimulant, so the cause likely isn't nutritional. That leaves one remaining option, emotional. You must have thought something that triggered a memory from your Unsafe Box. Now you are in a fight/flight mode, and your heart reacts accordingly. In April's case, it was a family conflict.

Often, a patient's symptoms disappear quickly once he or she understands the reason. It wasn't that easy for April. Though her symptoms seemed to come out of nowhere, there had to be a cause. The family conflict she was thinking about related to memories of many other conflicts. It took a lot of thought and introspection to work through her thoughts and memories. As she came to view her rapid heart rate episodes as teaching moments, she learned how to look at and respond to conflicts differently. It took many months for her to learn how to do this. Now her heart related symptoms are very rare, and she knows where they come from and what to do.

Here is our main objective in order to have good physical health.

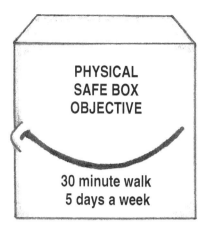

THE PHYSICAL ADD TWO PLAN

If you are really out of shape, or just can't find the time to exercise, I suggest the *Physical Add Two Plan*. Walk 2 minutes a day Monday through Friday for one week. The next week add 2 more minutes to your daily walk. Keep adding 2 minutes a week to your daily walk until you are walking 30 minutes a day 5 days a week. Two minutes isn't hard to find. Park farther away at the grocery store, walk up the stairs at work; find some excuse to walk a little extra. It's well worth the effort.

Samuel stepped in a hole and twisted his foot. It gradually improved over the next two months, but never completely healed. There was always some pain.

We treated Samuel and worked on some possible emotional stress, but he still didn't improve. After six months Samuel decided he needed to start walking for exercise. His foot hurt as he started walking, so he started out slowly and didn't walk very far. But it felt better at the end of his walk than it did at the beginning. So he walked the next day. After walking six days in a row, Samuel said to me, *"The pain in my foot is 75 percent gone. I can't believe how much better it feels from walking!"*

Samuel's foot had healed. It just needed some therapy to get the blood flowing and the muscles and tendons loosened up.

There is a simple principle here we need to emphasize in relation to injuries and exercise:

§ **If the pain gets less as you walk or exercise, then you need to exercise.**

§ **If the pain gets worse as you walk or exercise, then you are not yet ready to exercise.**

Sometimes we just need to exercise our body more to get well. You do need to give your body time to heal, but exercise is the best thing you can do when the time is right.

WALKING'S BONUS BENEFITS

Exercise is important, but there is another excellent reason to walk or do some other similar activity. Jim said, *"I usually walk at least five days a week. But I do it for more than the exercise. It is a sorting out time for me. It is a time to think, ponder, and solve problems. Most of my inspiration comes in the morning when I walk."*

Like Jim, we all need a time to think, ponder and sort out our lives. Going for a walk, even on a tread mill, can provide unimpeded, uninterrupted, and undisturbed time to think. During a mild exercise like this, you are doing two important things at once, exerting your body physically and your mind mentally.

Jim also added, *"I have learned that if I think too much about problems while I walk, my back will start to tighten up. If I think about solutions, I can get my back to relax and the pain goes away."* Walking has helped Jim recognize how his mind and body work together and how he has control over that. It is bonus benefit he did not expect.

Jim reminds us that what we think about we bring about, that if we are living in faith rather than in fear we physically feel better. A walk is not just good physical therapy. It is also good mental and emotional exercise.

This simple exercise routine of walking 30 minutes a day should become an invigorating and rejuvenating experience, one you look forward to as much for the mental and emotional benefits as the physical.

Part 2

3 STEPS TO HEAL YOURSELF

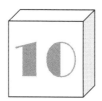

3 STEPS TO HEALING

You should now have a much better understanding of how and why symptoms develop, and what it really is that makes you sick. Hopefully you have even learned some of the true physical, nutritional and emotional causes of the symptoms you have, and have started to fix them. In this section we are going to discuss what you need to do to continue to heal and get well.

Refer back to the symptoms you listed in Chapter 1 and see if you have any different thoughts about them now. Do you better understand why you have them? Do you know the cause of any of them? Would you rate any of them differently now than you did then? Do you have any more that you would like to add to the list?

If you know the cause of your symptoms, you can find their solution. What a great blessing that can be! If you don't know the cause, then you have likely experienced some terrible frustration looking for relief. That will be the situation for the typical person who reads this book. In this section we will show you some ways to find the causes, and give you suggestions of how to fix the problems. As you apply the steps of healing, wellness will be the natural result.

We have two objectives in this section of the book.

1. **To help you eliminate known symptoms.**
2. **To help you establish a pattern of wellness so symptoms are not necessary.**

IDENTIFYING THE CAUSE

Let's take a fairly typical example of someone who has a reason to apply this program of healing and wellness. Pamela's immediate concern is her back. She typically walks one mile a day for exercise, and had just walked that mile and was feeling fine. She sat down to tie her shoes, and got a sudden pain in her back when she tried to stand up. It is now difficult for her to walk or sit. She has also had high blood pressure for 20 years, and had a heart attack 10 years ago. She has been in publishing for 25 years, and has daily deadlines at work, which is always stressful for her. She has a family situation that has been less than ideal for most of her marriage. She is 30 pounds over weight. She started eating a little better than the average person after her heart attack.

We had Pamela fill in the following chart to help identify the cause of her symptoms. We asked her to list her symptoms, when they started, and the possible physical, nutritional, and emotional causes. Here is how Pam completed her chart.

Symptom	Emotional Cause	Nutritional Cause	Physical Cause	When Started
Back pain	Don't know	Don't know	Tying shoes	Today
High Blood Pressure	Work? Family?	Probably weight	Not enough exercise	15-20 years ago
Heart Attack	Work? Family?	Poor diet	Not enough exercise	10 years ago
Over Weight	Don't know	Diet not adequate	Not enough exercise	30 years ago

You can see that Pam was quite uncertain about any emotional causes of her symptoms, had a better understanding about nutritional causes, and an even greater understanding of physical causes. This type of chart is useful in trying to identify the physical, nutritional and emotional causes of one's symptoms.

There are three observations we generally see when we ask someone to fill out this chart.

1. The most common **physical cause** of a symptom is an injury or not enough exercise. Everyone typically understands this and nine out of ten people (my observation) know what to do about it. They know what to do to recover from the injury or which exercise would help.

2. The most common **nutritional cause** is the diet is not good enough, meaning too much junk food and not enough fruits, vegetables, whole grains, etc. More and more people are aware of this, yet most are not able to connect it to their health. Three out of ten people (my observation) have a general idea what to do about it and about one out of ten know specifically what to do to improve.

3. The most common **emotional cause** is unknown or vague. In fact, most people don't even consider this in connection to their health. Of those who do, maybe one in twenty (my observation) have a general idea what to do about it. Maybe half of those know what to do to improve.

Pam knows there is stress at work and in her family, but she doesn't know exactly what "stress" means, or what the solution is. She just lives with it. Like the average person, she does not consider emotions as the cause of her symptoms. Yet of Pam's four complaints listed above, the emotional cause is the most important one to work on.

So what does Pam need to do to get well?

1. **Physical** - She needs to exercise more, though she is doing well to walk a mile a day. Increasing her daily walk to two miles a day, five days a week would be beneficial, though would probably provide only 5% - 10% improvement in her health.

2. **Nutritional** - She has made significant dietary changes since her heart attack, and at least eats some fruits, vegetables and whole grains now. But she needs to eat even more of those foods. She also needs to cut back on sweets and protein and strive harder for a diet that is 75% alkaline ash. By doing so she would likely see a 20% - 30% improvement in her health, depending on the degree of change.

3. **Emotional** - Pam's back went out because of the stress she was thinking about as she walked. It "weighed" too much. All she had to do was bend over, and as the familiar expression says, it was the final "straw that broke the camel's back." Her chronic high blood pressure and heart attack were classic examples of the effects of stress. By learning how to live in the Safe Box rather than the Unsafe Box, she could likely see a 60% - 70% improvement in her health. She needed a lot of understanding and help in this area to truly heal, be well, and prevent future health problems.

As we help Pamela recognize emotional causes it is also important to remember our premise from the beginning – there is nothing more magnificent on the earth than the human body. It never makes a mistake, and does everything it does for a reason. Letting go, seeing things through an eye of faith rather than fear, and making proper choices in the three areas above allows us to heal and be well.

Here are the 3 steps that Pamela and all of us need to do to heal and be well.

3 STEPS TO HEALING AND WELLNESS

STEP 1. EMOTIONAL CHOICES
Take all memories, thoughts, feelings, and stresses out of the Unsafe Box and put them in the Safe Box.

STEP 2. NUTRITIONAL CHOICES
Eat a diet that is 75% alkaline ash, and 25% acid ash.

STEP 3. PHYSICAL CHOICES
Take a brisk 30 minute walk 5 days a week (or something comparable).

Don't let this seem impossible or overwhelming. To get started, use the *Add Two Plan* for each of these 3 Steps. They've been mentioned before, but here they are, all together, to help you get started.

3 STEPS TO HEALING AND WELLNESS
The Add 2 Plan

STEP 1. EMOTIONAL CHOICES
GOAL - Take all memories, thoughts, feelings, and stresses out of the Unsafe Box and put in the Safe Box.

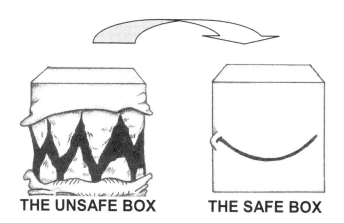

THE UNSAFE BOX　　　**THE SAFE BOX**

The Emotional Add 2 Plan

Take 2 negative situations, experiences or memories out of your Unsafe Box and add them to your Safe Box. Work on those for a day, being grateful they are as good as they are, letting go, forgiving and seeing God's hand in them (if that fits your beliefs). The next day add 2 more stressful situations or experiences to your Safe Box, and work on those for a day. Continue to Add 2 stresses or memories to your Safe Box each day, until your Unsafe Box is empty. This is a powerful mental and emotional exercise. Dealing with everything stored as Unsafe, and using all of this positive thinking to make it Safe, will have a powerful effect on your life.

STEP 2. NUTRITIONAL CHOICES
GOAL - Eat a diet that is 75% alkaline ash, and 25% acid ash.

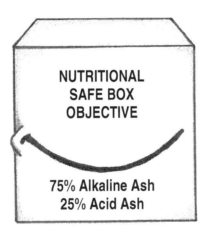

The Nutritional Add 2 Plan

Add 2 fruits, 2 vegetables and 2 glasses of water to your daily diet for a week in addition to what you normally consume. If you handle that well, without any cleansing symptoms, then add 2 more servings for another week. Repeat that until you are eating 75 percent alkaline ash foods. (If you develop cleansing symptoms like a skin rash, headaches, upset stomach, runny nose, etc., cut back on the fruit until symptoms disappear, then increase the fruit again.)

STEP 3. PHYSICAL CHOICES

GOAL - Take a brisk 30 minute walk 5 days a week (or something comparable).

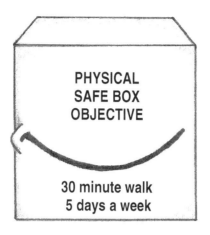

THE PHYSICAL ADD 2 PLAN

If you can't walk for 30 minutes because of physical or time limitations, start out slowly. Walk 2 minutes a day Monday through Friday for one week. The next week add 2 more minutes to your daily walk. Keep adding 2 minutes a week to your daily walk until you are walking 30 minutes a day 5 days a week.

CHART OF PROGRESS

It often helps to monitor the progress you are making. Set some goals for a month and use the chart on the following page to help track your efforts. Notice how your symptoms are affected as you make changes.

DAY	STEP 1. LIST 2 STRESSES OR MEMORIES ADDED TO SAFE BOX	STEP 2. LIST 2 EXTRA FRUITS AND VEGETABLES EATEN	STEP 3. LIST TIME EXERCISED
WK 1 MON			
TUE			
WED			
THU			
FRI			
SAT			
SUN			
WK 2 MON			
TUE			
WED			
THU			
FRI			
SAT			
SUN			
WK 3 MON			
TUE			
WED			
THU			
FRI			
SAT			
SUN			
WK 4 MON			
TUE			
WED			
THU			
FRI			
SAT			
SUN			

ADD 2 PLAN PROGRESS CHART

These 3 Steps to Healing are a simple outline of choices we need to make to be healthy. Step 1 is typically the most difficult, Step 2 typically easier, and Step 3 is usually the easiest.

In order to heal and be well, it important that we work on the step that is the cause. In most cases, all 3 steps are involved and all 3 need to be worked on. You should now have a good idea of how to apply Steps 2 and 3, the nutritional and physical steps, so we encourage you to go to work on them. Since Step 1 is generally the most important as well as the most difficult to identify and fix, the remaining chapters in this section are on how to identify and fix emotional causes of our symptoms.

IDENTIFYING EMOTIONAL CAUSES

Let's look again at Pamela's list of the emotional causes of her symptoms.

Symptom	Emotional Cause
Back pain	Don't know
High Blood Pressure	Work? Family?
Heart Attack	Work? Family?
Over Weight	Don't know

In order for Pam to do anything to heal or improve any of these symptoms resulting from emotional stress, she needs to have a much better understanding of what caused them. Remember that these causes are anything that makes Pam feel unsafe. Her heart attack happened ten years ago, and there may still be some things that Pamela needs to change to keep it from happening again. She is starting to work on the physical and nutritional things that affected her. Once she understands the emotional causes, she can then work on fixing them too. Her goal is to move any thoughts, feelings and memories from her

Emotional Unsafe Box into her Emotional Safe Box.

There are many ways a person can identify what the emotions are that are causing his symptoms. We will call them Emotional Identifiers and discuss the main ones. You may use any or all of the Emotional Identifiers, depending on how many symptoms you have and what works for you. Each one allows you to look at the cause of your symptoms a little differently. However, these Emotional Identifiers overlap and you may find a cause of your symptoms showing up in more than one. That simply reinforces what you need to work on.

EMOTIONAL IDENTIFIERS
1. *Current Stress*
2. *When Symptoms Began*
3. *Vivid memories*
4. *Undesirable Events*
5. *Unresolved Situations*
6. *Muscle Testing*

In the following chapters I will explain each Emotional Identifier on the list, what it means, how it works, and give an example of its use.

EMOTIONAL IDENTIFIER #1: CURRENT STRESS

Write in the Unsafe Box any current stresses that you have been thinking about, or that have been weighing on you, and any possible related symptoms.

UNSAFE BOX OF CURRENT STRESS	
Current Stresses	Possible Related Symptoms

What it means:

Anything we think about can be a stress. Deciding what to have for lunch is a stress, though a minor one. Planning meals for a family reunion is a stress, a more major one. If you go to bed with something on your mind, and wake up with it on your mind, and continue to do that day after day, you will eventually have some kind of physical symptom. If you think about the same stress many times a day, for many days, eventually some kind of physical symptom will show up.

Current stress often is the cause of current or recent symptoms. If your symptoms have been present for less than 3 months, there is likely a current stress that is a contributor.

How it works:

Stress turns on our fight/flight survival response. Muscles tense up, heart rate and blood pressure increase. Digestion slows down and sleep is more difficult. We get ready to run or fight. If we are in that mode too long, or too intensely, a variety of symptoms soon show up.

We think in order to solve and create, or defend and protect. If we solve quickly, like with what to have for lunch, that stress is over quickly, and it has no impact. If your family reunion is two months away, and you worry about it every day, there is a good chance you are going to get sick. Thinking about something too intensely for too long a period of time keeps our fight / flight survival response turned on too long, and eventually we have physical problems.

Hints Current Stress is a cause:

1. If you don't know what you did to bring on the symptoms, stress is a likely cause.
2. If you should be getting better faster than you are, stress is probably involved.
3. If you are not healing from an injury or surgery, consider stress as a factor.
4. If you say, *"I hurt, but I didn't do anything,"* it is likely stress related. (If stress is not the culprit, then you will need to look at your nutrition.)

Example 1:

Pamela, who we talked about earlier, had two huge deadlines coming up. She had projects she needed to get done, and she was behind schedule. She had been putting in longer hours than usual at work. She was out walking for exercise, and thinking about the projects weighing on her. She sat down to tie her shoe, and her back went out.

Pamela was stressed, both day and night. Her mind was constantly going, worrying about her deadlines. The muscles in her back were too tense for too long and overloaded from the stress. The little strain of bending over pulled her vertebra out of alignment. She came to our office for relief. By applying the reprogramming principles and addressing the cause of her problem immediately, she was able to get her muscles to quickly relax, and was 80% better the following day.

Example 2:

Carlos' neck had been hurting for about three months. He didn't know what brought it on, and it was not going away. In fact it seemed to be getting worse. Two months earlier Carlos' daughter got married. Though this was a happy occasion, Carlos was also sad. He was wondering how he would get along without his daughter around. They had been very close, and everything he had done had been for her. It almost seemed like a death in the family to him, rather than a celebration.

These were "unsafe" thoughts to Carlos, and his body reacted accordingly. Forgiving himself, being happy for his daughter, and applying other "reprogramming" steps had Carlos back to normal in a week.

Reprogramming Current Stress:

Now make the mental and emotional changes necessary to let go, or feel safe about these stressful things. This can happen quickly or take a lot of work and time, depending on the intensity of your feelings, and how easy it is to let go and see things differently.

Apply thoughts like the following to each stress you have listed in order to "reprogram" it and feel differently about it. You may come up with others that resonate with you better or fit your beliefs better. You need to feel what you are saying or thinking for it to have a positive physical impact. It needs to ring true, though it may take effort to see it that way. You may think these thoughts at any time, but it is ideal when you are quiet and reflective.

§ *I am grateful things are as good as they are.*

§ *I am grateful things aren't any worse, as they could be.*

§ *I forgive others for what they have done or said.*

§ *I forgive myself for how I have reacted and for how I have let it affect me.*

§ *I am grateful to see God's guiding and protecting hand in this.*

§ *I am grateful for the lesson of _____ I am learning from this.*

When you are able to feel safe about these Current Stresses, write them in the Safe Box below with the lesson learned (such as "I am more patient", "I am less judgmental", "I am more kind", "I've become more tolerant", etc).

SAFE BOX OF CURRENT STRESS	
Current Stresses	Lessons Learned

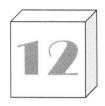

EMOTIONAL IDENTIFIER #2:
WHEN SYMPTOMS BEGAN

Write down your symptoms, when they began, and the possible situations or experiences that caused them.

UNSAFE BOX OF WHEN SYMPTOMS BEGAN		
Symptoms	When Began	Caused By

What it means:

The time a symptom begins is a good indicator of when stress reaches a critical point and starts to manifest itself physically. When Pamela's back goes out today, she should ask herself what she has been thinking about. She should also think of the stress she was under when she had her heart attack ten years ago. Carlos should wonder what was stressful to him three months ago when his neck pain first started. The symptom may manifest suddenly or gradually. So you can use the time the symptom first started as a very helpful emotional identifier.

How it works:

If we put more water into a bucket than it can hold, it spills over. Likewise, when the duration and/or intensity of the stress of a situation or incident reach a spillover or threshold point within us, symptoms become obvious.

Hints to understanding When Symptoms Began:
1. Ask yourself, *"What was going on in my life when this symptom started?"*
2. Ask yourself, *"Where was I living?*
3. Ask your self, *"What stage of life was I in?"*
4. Ask yourself, *"How old was I at the time?"*

Example 1:

Fatigue had been a problem for Naomi for about twenty years. She had been diagnosed with adrenal insufficiency at age fifteen and had been taking steroid medication since.

The medication helped her function so she wasn't totally exhausted. To identify the *cause* of her fatigue, Naomi should ask herself, *"What happened at age fifteen?"*

Naomi remembered that she would come home after school, go to bed, eat supper, and go back to bed. She could sleep all the time. What was the stress? It was about then that her mother got sick. Naomi remembered being in a hospital room with her mother, when the doctor came in and showed a chart, explaining her mother possibly had AIDS or some other serious illness. Naomi said she felt "deflated". She knew from then on life would not be simple any more.

Naomi's feeling of being "deflated," physically deflated her. It took the wind out of her sails. It took the life out of her. Naomi needed to rethink that experience, and reprogram it differently. She needed to forgive herself for her reaction at the time and be grateful things were as good as they were and not any worse. As a result, her energy level significantly improved the next month and soon she was able to cut back on the steroids.

Example 2:

James had neck, back and arm pain and was chronically tired.

I asked James when it started and he said three years ago. So, of course my question was what happened three years ago? James said he went through a divorce. He was willing to work on the emotional causes, and in two weeks felt better than he had in three years.

Reprogramming When Symptoms Began:

Now you need to make the mental and emotional changes necessary to let go, or feel safe about these incidents or situations. Apply the same reprogramming we described earlier, ideally while in a quiet and reflective moment.

- § *I am grateful things are as good as they are.*
- § *I am grateful things aren't any worse, as they could be.*
- § *I forgive others for what they have done or said.*
- § *I forgive myself for how I have reacted and for how I have let it affect me.*
- § *I am grateful to see God's guiding and protecting hand in this.*
- § *I am grateful for the lesson of _____ I am learning from this.*

When you are able to feel safe about these stressful experiences, write them in the Safe Box below with the lesson learned.

SAFE BOX OF WHEN SYMPTOMS BEGAN	
Cause of Symptoms	Lessons Learned

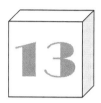

EMOTIONAL IDENTIFIER #3: VIVID MEMORIES

Write down any vivid memories you have, your age at the time and possible symptoms associated with them, if you can think of any.

UNSAFE BOX OF VIVID MEMORIES		
Vivid Memories	Age	Possible Symptoms

What it means:

In the vivid memories are often lessons to be learned. When we can remember specific words said or thoughts thought, there is a lesson. When we can picture a memory in living color with full detail, and even have smells come back to us, there is a purpose for that memory. As we said in Chapter 7, Renee having a vivid picture in her mind of her sister being thrown against the wall, Harold having a vivid memory sitting in his desk at kindergarten, and Judy not wanting to re-visit what happened at age six were all teachers of important life lessons. These memories often have some type of symptom tied to them. They definitely influence our perception of life.

How it works:

The vivid memory usually flies in the face of what we expect, consciously or even subconsciously. There is typically something extremely incongruent about it. It is physically or emotionally threatening. We don't know how to interpret it, based on the perceptions we have. Other life experiences that fit within our expectations seem to be filed neatly away in our "computer's" memory. But the vivid ones don't have a place to go. We don't have a file folder for them. They don't add up, don't make sense, and stay in our "In Box" waiting to be handled. They need to be processed. They are in our Unsafe Box and need to be moved to the Safe Box.

Hints to understanding Vivid Memories:

Reflect on various stages or ages of your life, and see if a vivid memory comes to mind. You might think in terms of education, such as pre-school, elementary school, etc. or ages 0-5 years, 5-10 years, 10-15 years, etc.

Example 1:

Yvonne had a vivid memory of her childhood bedroom. It was the dugout space under their house where the furnace was located. Just thinking of it brought a musty odor to her senses, and she said, *"I can still smell it today."* In addition, if Yvonne went somewhere and smelled a musty smell, it would plug her up and she would have a difficult time breathing. Reprogramming that memory by making it safe allowed her to overcome her reaction to the odor.

Example 2:

Rod had an allergy to cats, so I asked him if he had a bad memory relating to cats. He most definitely did. He said he crawled under the bed when he was three years old and a cat jumped out at him and bit him on the lip. He said he could remember it as if it had happened yesterday, though it occurred more than 50 years earlier. He then said, *"I hate cats. I shoot them. After I shoot a cat, I go over to it and say, 'And you won't bite me in the mouth!'"*

Such a reaction tells us that Rod still has lots of feelings tied up in that experience as a three year old. Our discussion was quite enlightening to Rod as he had never recognized how his allergies could be tied in with this experience. I also found it quite interesting that Rod had hunted animals all over the world. His prize trophy, out of his entire big animal collection, was a female lion (a big cat), the *"wiliest of all animals to hunt"*. (A year after treating Rod I learned that he was off on another big hunt, after an animal even more cunning and dangerous than a female lion – a cheetah.)

Reprogramming Vivid Memories:

As we said before, make the mental and emotional changes necessary to feel safe about these Vivid Memories. Apply the same reprogramming we described earlier, ideally while in a quiet and reflective moment.

§ *I am grateful things are as good as they are.*
§ *I am grateful things aren't any worse, as they could be.*
§ *I forgive others for what they have done or said.*
§ *I forgive myself for how I have reacted and for how I have let it affect me.*
§ *I am grateful to see God's guiding and protecting hand in this.*
§ *I am grateful for the lesson of _____ I am learning from this.*

When you are able to feel safe about these Vivid Memories, write them in the Safe Box below with the lesson learned.

SAFE BOX OF VIVID MEMORIES	
Vivid Memories	Lessons Learned

EMOTIONAL IDENTIFIER #4: UNDESIRABLE EVENTS

Write down any unwanted or undesired events, your age at the time it occurred and possible symptoms associated with them, if you can think of any.

UNSAFE BOX OF UNDESIRABLE EVENTS		
Undesirable Event	Age	Possible Symptoms

What it means:

Undesirable Events are things that have happened that we wish hadn't happened or we wish had been different. We may not have a vivid memory attached to them, and may not recognize any symptom begun by them. Yet they can still be a source of fear or worry, and they can still influence our survival response and contribute to symptoms. They may be major things like divorce and death, or seemingly more minor things like failing a test or being embarrassed. They still end up in our Unsafe Box and are things we don't want to repeat.

How it works:
An event that happens to us that we wish hadn't happened or had been different is a threat to our physical or emotional safety. It doesn't match our expectation or perception of what should be, and creates a defensive reaction on the part of our body. Symptoms may be created if we feel intensely enough about it, or if that event is repeated. In fact many stressful experiences that cause symptoms have a previous Undesirable Event tied to them as we talked about in Chapter 6 under the *Law of Witnesses*. In order to heal and be well we need to reprogram both the stress that triggers the symptom and the similar Undesirable Events prior to it.

Hints to understanding Undesirable Events:
1. Consider the question, *What has happened in my life that I wish hadn't happened or had been different?*
2. Reflect on various stages or ages of your life, as we suggested in Vivid Memories, and see if an Undesirable Event comes to mind.
3. If you have been able to identify a stressful experience that was the cause of your symptoms, consider what undesired similar events might have happened previous to it, and add these to your list.

Example 1:
Raymond was an excellent student up to third grade. He loved to learn and believed he was the teacher's pet. Something happened in the bathroom at school one day that changed him. Raymond got in a fight with another boy and held the boy's arm against a hot water pipe, burning his arm. Raymond couldn't remember for sure what caused the fight, but thought it dad something to do with him being the teacher's favorite. Raymond didn't like school after that, and didn't do well. He struggled with friends and felt alone and unaccepted.

Though Raymond didn't develop any physical symptoms

from this incident, he recognized emotional ones. He had been emotionally injured, and knew that incident had changed his life. At age thirty he realized how this Undesirable Event was continuing to impact his life in the ways he dealt with people. He knew he had to get it out of his Unsafe Box and into his Safe Box if he was going to be the kind of person he wanted to be.

Example 2:

Marianne couldn't breathe through her nose. She had been that way for five months, no matter what she did.

Marianne's breathing problem started when her brother was killed in a motorcycle accident. So the obvious Emotional Identifier was When Symptoms Began, or her brother's death. But working on that wasn't enough to get her breathing through her nose again. She then told me of another Undesirable Event that happened several years earlier when two of her other brothers had crashed into each other, and one of them was killed. I asked if there was any one else she had been close to who had passed away, or another Undesirable Event, and she said *"her grandmother"*. After reprogramming those memories, Marianne was able to breathe through her nose the next day, and hasn't had a problem since.

Reprogramming Undesirable Events:

Make the mental and emotional changes necessary to feel safe about these Undesirable Events. Once again, apply the same reprogramming we described earlier, ideally while in a quiet and reflective moment.

§ *I am grateful things are as good as they are.*
§ *I am grateful things aren't any worse, as they could be.*
§ *I forgive others for what they have done or said.*
§ *I forgive myself for how I have reacted and for how I have let it affect me.*
§ *I am grateful to see God's guiding and protecting hand in this.*
§ *I am grateful for the lesson of _____ I am learning from this.*

.When you are able to feel safe about these Undesirable Events, write them in the Safe Box below with the lesson learned.

SAFE BOX OF UNDESIRABLE EVENTS	
Undesirable Events	Lessons Learned

EMOTIONAL IDENTIFIER #5: UNRESOLVED SITUATIONS

Write down any current or past situations that you feel are unresolved, whether or not you can do anything about them, and any possible related symptoms.

UNSAFE BOX OF UNRESOLVED SITUATIONS		
Unresolved Situations	Current or Past	Possible Symptoms

What it means:

Unresolved Situations leave us hanging. They are situations where the outcome has not been decided, or decided to our satisfaction. We feel the ball is still in our court or someone else's court, and the game is not yet over. Like hanging over the edge of a cliff, Unresolved Situations can be frightening, depending on their size. They may be things from the past or from the present. If situations are left hanging, or unresolved, they are a threat to us, and we will eventually develop symptoms.

How it works:
An Unresolved Situation does not have an end to it, so we are still waiting for the outcome. We are still waiting for closure. Our Initial Judgment is that it is unsafe, and it will remain in our Unsafe Box until we can bring closure to it. Like Vivid Memories, Unresolved Situations wait for an end in order to be filed in our "computer". If they exist long enough, or if we feel them intensely enough, they will create physical symptoms like exhaustion, difficulty sleeping, digestive problems, and other symptoms we have talked about. Present Unresolved Situations are especially difficult to deal with because of the real fear they could get worse.

Hints to understanding Unresolved Situations:
1. Think of any *present* Unresolved Situations dealing with family, school, work, church, friends, etc.
2. Think of any *past* Unresolved Situations dealing with family, school, work, church, friends, etc.
3. Are you in a situation you are afraid will not improve, or a situation which might even get worse?

Again, it is helpful to consider the various ages and stages of your life.

Example 1:
Shelly had back pain, headaches, poor digestion, allergies, and insomnia.

Shelly's Unresolved Situation had to do with her father-in-law. They were next door neighbors, but as a result of a conflict, had not spoken to each other for two years. For six months Shelly had been feeling she needed to talk to him and try to mend things. But she just couldn't get up the nerve to do it. She finally decided a certain Sunday would be the day she would approach him. The Saturday before, he had a heart attack and passed away. She felt a horrible guilt for not having made amends with him, and now she felt there was no possible way to do so. But how could she live with the guilt?

Even in a circumstance like Shelly's, there is a way to be free of the burden. As with each of the Emotional Identifiers, the approach will vary depending on one's beliefs. Shelly found relief through repentance and forgiveness in prayer. Her faith was such that prayer was the ideal solution for her. (Writing a letter to the father-in-law, as if he was alive, or talking to the mother-in-law may be the right solution for someone else.) Shelly had a wonderful healing experience. She was at peace again, and her symptoms all improved.

Example 2:

Cody did some subcontracting for various general contractors. One of his competitors did not appreciate losing work to Cody so he repeatedly filed law suits against him. Cody spent lots of money and time defending himself in court. He came to see me with pain in his leg, which always flared up when he was dealing with his legal dilemma.

We treated Cody and could help him some, but letting go and being grateful are not easy to do when you fear you are likely to be sued again. His Unresolved Situation made it very difficult for him to continue to stay well. It required a great deal of emotional and mental effort for Cody to successfully deal with his ongoing situation. Though it was difficult, Cody knew that when his leg flared up, he again had some forgiving and letting go to do.

Reprogramming Unresolved Situations:

Make the mental and emotional changes necessary to feel safe about these Unresolved Situations. Apply the same reprogramming we described earlier, ideally while in a quiet and reflective moment.

§ *I am grateful things are as good as they are.*
§ *I am grateful things aren't any worse, as they could be.*
§ *I forgive others for what they have done or said.*
§ *I forgive myself for how I have reacted and for how I*

have let it affect me.

§   *I am grateful to see God's guiding and protecting hand in this.*

§   *I am grateful for the lesson of _____ I am learning from this.*

When you are able to feel safe about these Unresolved Situations, write them in the Safe Box below with the lesson learned.

SAFE BOX OF UNRESOLVED SITUATIONS	
Unresolved Situations	Lessons Learned

EMOTIONAL IDENTIFIER #6: MUSCLE TESTING

We now need to explain muscle testing, a very useful tool that may help you in your healing process, and can be used with each of the Emotional Identifiers we have already discussed. Muscle testing has been used by many practitioners for many years to help identify the body's response to a variety of things. It has increased in popularity and is used in coaching and education and many other ways. In fact, there is a good chance that you have had muscle testing done on you, or even have done it yourself.

Muscle testing is a major technique we use in our office to identify emotional causes of symptoms. It is a powerful and simple tool and we encourage its use. I must emphasize, however, that it is just an emotional identifier, and is not necessary to heal or be well. So you do not need to use it. Its main advantage is that you can more specifically identify what is in your Unsafe Box, as well as confirm what you have put in the Safe Box. The instructions on the following pages tell you how to perform a muscle test with a partner. It can take some practice to get comfortable with it, and you should know that some people are easier to test than others. But it is a great tool, and could make a huge difference in understanding and solving your health problems

You will need to have someone assist you with this test, having him or her press against your arm while you are thinking of different thoughts. We will explain the specifics a little later, but generally speaking, your strong arm will stay strong when you think of a safe experience. It will go weaker when you think of an unsafe experience. We have mentioned many times how a thought will affect the body. Though we have typically talked about that in the terms of how a thought can make a person sick, we can also use it in an intentional way to see the effect of a thought on the body.

We can compare the muscle test to the response felt when pushing down on a table top, or pushing down on a balloon that is on the table top. A "strong arm" is like pushing on the table top. There is an immediate and firm response. A "weak arm" is like pushing on the balloon. There is a softer, slower, more sluggish response.

For example, suppose you suffer with an injury from a car accident three years ago. The accident is not a good memory for you. You have a friend gently muscle test your right arm while you are thinking of a pleasant thought, such as a sunset or mountain scene. He finds your arm responds firmly and immediately. It is "strong" like pushing down on the table top. You then think of the accident, and have him test the arm again. This time it is "weak" like pushing down on the balloon. It doesn't respond as fast. It feels sluggish or mushy to him. That means that thought is "unsafe". You react to it when you think of it, and there is a physical impact on your body causing your arm to go weaker.

The body's number one instinct is to survive. When you think of the accident, it triggers a defensive reaction on the part of the body. All systems go on alert as you don't want to repeat that experience again. When your friend pushes on your arm while you think of the accident, your brain essentially says, *"Ignore the arm! We have a potential emergency here!"* So the split second it normally takes you to respond when thinking of the pleasant thought, now takes three or four split seconds when you think of the accident. So we say the arm is "weak". The muscle test allows you to identify how your body responds to a stress or memory. It is a subconscious reaction based on previous experiences. Your conscious perception of the stress or memory can be much different than your subconscious one. In fact, that is often the case and a reason a person fails to heal or get well.

Once the memory of the accident is identified as a **cause** of why your body will not heal, you can then fix the memory. You can choose to see it differently. You can move it from your Unsafe Box into your Safe Box. You can be grateful that you survived. You can be grateful it wasn't any worse. You can see God's hand in it and learn a lesson of forgiveness toward others involved, and even yourself.

When you feel that you have been able to move the memory into the Safe Box, you can now think of the accident again, and have your friend muscle test you once more. This time, if you were able to get the memory in the Safe Box like you thought you did, the arm will respond immediately. It will be "strong". If your arm stays "weak", then you weren't able to shift the memory into the Safe Box for reasons which we will describe later.

HOW TO MUSCLE TEST

Here are the steps to muscle testing. I will describe them as if you are helping your friend by doing the testing.

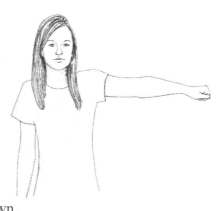

1. Stand behind your partner with him looking straight ahead. Have him hold his dominant arm straight out to the side with hand open and palm down.
2. Place your hand on his wrist and your opposite hand on his opposite shoulder for stability.
3. Ask your partner to hold his arm still, resisting while you press gently but firmly down on his wrist toward the floor. His arm should be "strong" like pushing down on

the table top. (If his arm does not respond immediately, test his other arm, and use the one that responds the best.)

4. Have your partner think of a pleasant thought, such as a sunrise or holding a baby, and test his arm again. It should remain "strong".

5. Now have your partner think of something that is stressful or of a bad experience while you re-test his arm. If his arm goes "weak" like pushing down on the balloon on the table top, then you have an unsafe thought.

6. Have him fix the unsafe thought by doing what he needs to put it in his Safe Box. That means seeing it differently by being grateful, forgiving, and letting go.

7. Have him think again of the unsafe thought while muscle testing his arm. This time his arm should be "strong".

Reprogramming with Muscle Testing:

Once you understand the above procedure, you can begin to use muscle testing to help identify and treat the cause of your symptoms. Symptoms, as we have discussed, can come from current stresses or memories of past experiences that are stored in our Unsafe Box. We want to make those safe. We should note that some memories are known, and some are forgotten or hidden. With muscle testing we can even identify the hidden ones that might be affecting us, and make those safe as well.

So the goal of our muscle testing is this:

Objective 1 - Identify a stress or memory that makes the arm go WEAK when thought of.

Objective 2 - Fix that stress or memory so the arm stays STRONG when thought of.

This is important, so let me repeat it. Find a thought that makes the arm go weak. Fix the thought and the arm will be strong. Objective 1 is a weak arm. Objective 2 is a strong arm.

Example 1:

Jana's left elbow has hurt for four months, and isn't getting any better. She thinks she may have strained it lifting her grand-daughter, but doesn't remember a specific incident. She wants to apply some of the things we have talked about to see if it will help her. Because it started four months ago, and hasn't improved, she tries to remember something stressful going on at that time. She has her sister muscle test her to identify the cause in order to achieve Objectives 1 and 2 above. Here are the steps that Jana follows:

Objective 1 -

1. Jana thinks of a beautiful sunrise and her sister tests her arm. It is strong. She knows she responds favorably to a positive thought.

2. Jana thinks her stress four months earlier may have been that her grand-daughter was visiting for only a short time, and Jana had to work. She felt bad that she was working and she was torn with feelings as to where she should really be. As she thinks of this memory, her sister again tests her arm. It is weak. She has now achieved Objective 1. She has identified the stress that makes her arm go weak.

Objective 2 -

1. Jana lets go of the experience in her mind and sees it differently. She reflects on how grateful she is that she does have a job, that her grand-daughter came, and that she was able to spend as much time with her as she did. She forgives herself for being so negative and critical of herself. She moves her memory from her Unsafe Box to her Safe Box.

2. Now Jana thinks of the stressful situation again, and her sister tests her arm once more. This time her arm stays strong, and does not go weak like it did before. She now has achieved Objective 2. She has fixed the stress that made her arm go weak. She has moved that memory from her Unsafe Box to her Safe Box. Her body will now begin to heal and her elbow should improve.

If Jana's elbow does not improve, then she was either not

able to maintain her memory of four months earlier in her Safe Box, or there was an additional cause involved. We should note that the benefit of muscle testing is that it helped Jana identify the stress that was affecting her. Pinpointing the one that made her arm go weak means she is working on a cause. There could be more than one cause, and Jana could also have her sister test her for others she thinks might be involved.

Example 2:

Krystal had had extremely dry eyes for ten years. They were always red and burned and itched all the time. Her ophthalmologist said they were the worst case he had ever seen.

Objective 1 –

Krystal's first objective with muscle testing is to find something she thinks of that makes her arm go weak. Applying the "Emotional Identifier of When Symptoms Began", she thought back to ten years ago when her symptoms first started. She got pregnant back then, and her boyfriend left her. About that experience she said, *"I cried for a long time. I finally decided that crying didn't help, and I would not cry any more."* She was successful with that "goal" and literally had not cried since. She could hardly even make a tear, and thus the dry eyes. When she thought of that memory, her arm tested weak, so she had achieved Objective 1.

Objective 2 –

Krystal's second objective was for her arm to remain strong when she thought of that Undesirable Event in her life. So she went through the forgiveness and letting go process. When she was muscle tested again, while thinking of her former boyfriend, this time her arm remained strong. So she had done what she needed to do to take that memory out of her Unsafe Box and put it in her Safe Box.

Though Krystal was able to successfully put that memory in her Safe Box, it did not stay there very easily. She had to work on the forgiving and letting go several times as it was such a painful memory. Her eyes improved about 75 percent, and she could actually get tears in her eyes.

A few months later Krystal's eyes got worse again. What was the cause?

Occasionally something comes up that triggers symptoms again. It has to be something emotionally threatening enough to pull the memory out of the Safe Box and put it back into the Unsafe Box. Krystal thought it would be good if she was muscle tested again.

Objective 1 –

Krystal's dry eyes began with a boyfriend problem, so it would be logical to wonder if the cause was another boyfriend problem. Krystal said her current boyfriend lived four hundred miles away and was trying to sell his business so he could move to be with her. When Krystal thought of her current boyfriend, her arm tested weak, indicating she had found the probable cause of her eyes becoming worse.

Objective 2 –

As much as Krystal wanted her boyfriend to move and be with her, it was a frightening thought based on past experience. That memory was not something she wanted to repeat. In order to feel safe Krystal had to forgive and let go once again of the past. She had to let go of the present fear that this boy friend would leave too. She needed to have faith that all would be well, no matter the outcome. Then when she thought of her current boyfriend her arm tested strong, confirming that she had put the past memory and the current fear in her Safe Box where they needed to be. Within a couple of days her eyes were much better again.

Example 3:

Let's take someone whose story is a little more complicated, and see how muscle testing could help identify the cause of her symptoms and help her heal and get well. Claire was fifty years old.

This was some of Claire's background – She spent much of her early childhood in a bar because that is where her parents were. By the time she was five, she was often responsible for younger siblings. She injured her back in a horse accident in high school and her neck in a car accident a few years later. Her son was killed in a car accident eight years earlier.

These were some of Claire's current stresses – Her son-in-law was a partner in their business and she and her husband had recently discovered he had stolen a significant amount of money from them. She had raised her ten year old grand-daughter since she was a baby. The girl's mother (Claire's daughter) and her husband had just moved in with them, but spent a lot of time at the bar. Claire was responsible for an immense amount of government paper work with their business, and she was not comfortable with it.

These were Claire's symptoms – Neck pain, migraine headaches (about six a year before her son died to three or four a week after he died), shoulder pain, low back pain, can't lay flat at night so sleeps sitting up, doesn't sleep well, dizziness, blurred vision, exhaustion, frequent nausea, hormonal problems and hand pain.

Claire also told me she'd had poor health most of her life. She had lived in pain as long as she could remember, and had been to two pain clinics in the past five years with little relief. She was taking ten prescription medications.

These were just some of the major things about Claire. In addition, she ate very little fruit and few vegetables, drank more soda pop than water, and did not exercise.

Though Claire had many symptoms, and had been given many diagnoses, there was much she could do for herself to be well. The easiest things were to start getting some exercise and eating better. Let's also consider the five Emotional Identifiers.

1. *Did her Unsafe Box of **Current Stress** have anything in it?*
2. *Did her Unsafe Box of **When Symptoms Began** have anything in it?*
3. *Did her Unsafe Box of **Vivid Memories** have anything in it?*
4. *Did her Unsafe Box of **Undesirable Events** have anything in it?*
5. *Did her Unsafe Box of **Unresolved Situations** have anything in it?*

From what we know, it is quite obvious that Claire had something in each of her Unsafe Boxes. In fact, she would tell you they were full and that is where she lived. She could easily have made a list of forty or fifty stresses or negative memories. In order to heal and be well, Claire needed to move those thoughts, feelings, memories, and stresses into her Safe Box. That whole process was very overwhelming for her, with the length of her list, and the need to change her perception of so many things.

I suggested to Claire that she should use the *Emotional Add Two Plan* to help her heal and be well. I suggested that each day she take two situations or experiences out of her Unsafe Box and add them to her Safe Box. By doing this she could slowly make the emotional changes that would allow her to heal and become well, without becoming overwhelmed or discouraged. She could use muscle testing to help her identify the thoughts she needed to work on, and confirm that she had successfully put them in her Safe Box. Some things, like dealing with the son-in-law who stole the money, she may have to repeatedly work on for a long period of time.

For example, Claire could start with the Unsafe Box of Current Stress and choose one stress out of it to move to her Safe Box. She could have someone muscle test her to see if it met Objective 1, making her arm go weak. Then she would forgive and let go and have someone muscle test her again to see if she met Objective 2, making her arm stay strong. If it was strong, then she would pick another stress and repeat the procedure. If her arm was still weak, then she would work some more on the letting go, until it stayed strong when being tested. Then she would pick another stress and repeat the procedure.

When Claire had identified and fixed those two stresses, she would be done for the day. The rest of the day, she would make sure she still felt "safe" about those stresses. She would continue to feel grateful they were as good as they were, see God's hand in them, and learn the lessons from them.

The next day, Claire could go to the Unsafe Box of When Symptoms Began and pick two of those memories. She would be muscle tested for those, until she met Objective 1 and Objective 2, and then work on those the rest of the day.

The third day, Claire could go to the Unsafe Box of Vivid Memories, pick two of those and add them to her Safe Box. Gradually, little by little, she would work through her list of forty or fifty items and move them from her Unsafe Box into her Safe Box. She would change. Her life would change and her health would improve. The *Emotional Add Two* plan is a wonderful way of using positive thinking and reprogramming to improve our lives and health. Claire has worked on this, and continues to work on this, and is experiencing many positive changes in her life.

HIDDEN MEMORIES

It is not only known stresses and known memories that affect a person, but hidden, buried and forgotten memories may contribute to symptoms as well. That is likely the case with Claire. So it was with Celine.

Celine had trouble with restless legs for many years. It was worse in the evening and especially at night.

From an emotional perspective, Celine was "running". Her fight/flight system was turned on and sitting or lying still in bed when a figurative bear is attacking is not safe, so the legs "run". Celine used the Emotional Identifiers to help her work through several possible causes of her restless legs. Several causes were identified. As a small child, her mother would have her hide behind the couch when the landlord came to collect the rent. She always felt afraid the landlord would see her. Another was when she was eight years old. She was trapped when a cave she and her brothers were digging collapsed on her. She got a little better by working on these, but not much. What else could be contributing to Celine's restless legs?

Often a hidden or forgotten memory is the cause of the body responding the way it is. These too can be discovered through muscle testing. Instead of testing a specific memory or stress that we can recall, we can test an age or stage in life. If there is a memory at that age or stage that is threatening to the body, the arm will go weak when that period of time is thought of, just like thinking of a known threat.

So when muscle testing Celine, I had her think of the first

ten years of her life. I asked her to picture or imagine those years and then tested her arm. I then had her think of ages ten to twenty and tested her, twenty to twenty-nine and tested her, and so on. If there was a bad memory or a bad experience in the decade she was thinking of, then her arm tested weak. If not, then it stayed strong. (I could also have tested stages of life, such as pre-school, elementary school, junior high school, and so on, looking for the stage that would make her arm go weak.) When I identified an age that made Celine's arm go weak, I asked if she could remember a negative experience from that time.

Celine's arm tested weak when I had her think of the first ten years of her life. I knew there was something from that period of time in her Unsafe Box that was still affecting her. She couldn't recall anything from that time in her life that she hadn't already worked on. I then had her think of the first five years, and then from ages six to ten. Her arm tested weak on the first five years, but not on ages six to ten. I then tested her as she thought of each year, one, two, three, four and five. Her arm tested weak at age five. I knew that Celine had a memory from age five that was still unsafe to her and was interfering with her health.

It took Celine a few minutes to try to recall where they lived and what was going on at that early time in her life. Finally, the light came on. A neighbor family had been gassed one night and all died in their sleep. Two days later her family nearly had the same experience, but her grandmother woke up in the middle of the night. They barely escaped alive. I had her think of that memory and again her arm went weak, achieving Objective 1.

Is it surprising that Celine had legs that didn't want to stay still at night? Can you see how she might even have had a subconscious fear of ever going to sleep?

Celine hadn't thought of that experience for many, many years. That doesn't mean that her body was not programmed to respond to it. As a five year old, she likely didn't understand what it meant to be gassed. She would have understood that her neighbors had died, and that her family had nearly had the same experience. She especially would have felt the emotional tension and stress of her parents and other family members as they dealt with these tragic and near tragic events for an extended period of time.

The important thing for Celine to know was that at age sixty-six she was still reacting to those memories from age five. She had been "programmed" to respond to them, so it was normal for her to react the way she did. There are many things she learned at a young age that she was still doing in the same way. A simple example is tying her shoes. Likewise, her body had been programmed to "run" when she went to sleep at age five, and she was still doing it the same way. The only thing that could change that program was to reprogram the memory that started it. At age sixty-six, Celine could learn to tie her shoes differently, if she wanted. Likewise, she could learn to go to sleep differently. I had Celine apply forgiveness, gratitude and other healing lessons in order to let go of and reprogram her memory from age five. After she did so, we tested her arm strength again as she thought of the memory, and this time her arm stayed strong. Objective 2 was met.

Working on this memory from age five helped Celine greatly with her symptoms. But she had to remind herself for many nights as she went to bed that she was safe. A sixty year programmed pattern can be difficult to overcome, even when the cause is recognized. Using the *Add Two Plan Progress Chart* in Chapter 12 and including nutritional and physical changes along with the emotional helped her to significantly improve as well.

Some hidden memories, like Celine's, can be remembered quite quickly when an age or stage of life is pinpointed. Some may not come to mind until later. Hope told me it was a couple of hours after she left our office before it dawned on her what had happened. We had muscle tested her and identified that something had happened at age forty, but she couldn't remember what it was. On the way home, she remembered that was when her daughter was run over. Her daughter was four years old at the time, but Hope had never tied that experience in with her own age, so it didn't easily come to mind. We had helped Hope with this memory before, but it was not an easy one to overcome, and there was more that needed to be done. Her daughter had fallen out of the tractor her husband was driving, and she was run over across her pelvis. Her pelvis was broken, but she had miraculously survived and recovered, and now six years later, she had no residual effects.

Hope knew it was an accident, and had forgiven her husband, and didn't have any hard feelings there. Yet, each time her daughter would go out and ride on the tractor, Hope couldn't help but fear it would happen again. In fact it was difficult for Hope to let her daughter be gone for very long anywhere. She would constantly think about her and wonder if she was safe. You won't be surprised to learn that Hope's major complaints were anxiety and fatigue. Like Celine, Hope had a lot of work to do to put her daughter in her Safe Box and leave her there.

We should note here that both Celine and Hope could remember what happened to them after we identified an age that made their arm test weak. That is not always the case. If a specific memory doesn't come to mind, as it didn't with Hope at first, then we can work on the memory generally. We can think of the age or stage and make it positive and safe by forgiving ourselves and others for whatever took place. Doing that can make a significant difference in how a person feels and the symptoms he or she has.

AN ADDITIONAL HINT

Here is another suggestion as you use muscle testing to help yourself or someone else heal and become well. It is not a necessary step, but one that may help you get better and quicker results.

When all the causes have been identified and fixed, your arm should test strong when you think of a symptom.

Think of a symptom while someone muscle tests your arm. If your arm tests weak then there is likely a stress or memory contributing to the symptom. Find a stress or memory as we have discussed, and fix it, and then think of the symptom and test your arm again. If it is still weak, then there is another stress or memory still contributing to it. Try to find another one and fix it as well. Keep doing that until your arm tests strong when thinking of your symptom. At that point you have likely dealt with the cause, and should improve from there.

Shelton had digestive problems for several years.

Overall Shelton had improved significantly after we started treating him. One day he came in and said his stomach had really been bothering him the past six days. It had started when they had gone to visit family. I muscle tested him while he thought of his stomach troubles, and his arm went weak. I asked him if there was anything stressful about visiting his family. He said his dad was remarrying, and his sister-in-law was having a very difficult time with the idea. I had him think about that stress. His arm went weak, so he fixed that and put it in the Safe Box, and then I had him think about his stomach troubles again. His arm was still weak.

Shelton's mother had died six years earlier and his dad had moved in with their family. Shelton had voluntarily taken on the responsibility of seeing that his dad was okay. Shelton thought of that stress and his arm tested weak, so he fixed that memory as well.

Again, he thought of his symptom and his arm still tested weak. I tested Shelton again for different ages and found that his arm went weak at age two. He didn't have a memory from then, but knew that his mother had been very sick with stomach troubles herself. We updated that memory, and once more I had him think of his stomach troubles. This time his arm tested strong. I then knew we had worked on those things that were contributing to his stomach pain the past six days. He quickly improved from there.

Muscle testing is a good way to identify emotional causes and symptoms. It has helped a great number of my patients and can be a great help in your search to understand the cause of your symptoms.

Let's review what we have learned about Muscle Testing, Emotional Identifier #6.

1. **Objective 1 – Identify a thought that makes the arm test weak.**
2. **Objective 2 – Identify a thought that makes the arm test strong.**
3. **Muscle testing helps identify hidden memories and stresses.**

4. **Muscle testing helps identify ages or stages when negative things occurred.**
5. **When all the causes have been identified and fixed, the arm should test strong when thinking of a symptom.**

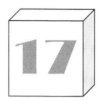

3 STEPS TO A
HEALTHY CHILD

As we talk about what we need to do to heal and be well, we eventually come to questions about our children. Their health is just as important, if not more so, than ours. What do we do for them? How do they fit in with the *3 Steps to Heal Yourself*?

Trends in children's health are troubling. Childhood obesity has increased significantly since 1980, more than tripling to almost 18 percent, and is still on the rise. Along with obesity come the related complications of diabetes and heart disease, also on the increase. (Recently, a patient told me her grand-daughter was just put on cholesterol lowering medication as her total cholesterol was 300 mg/dl – at age five!) Then there are allergies, asthma, ADHD, cancer and many other conditions that seem to be more prevalent. How much of this is avoidable, preventable and even reversible?

Let's look again at our 3 Steps to Healing and Wellness. How do they apply to children and their health?

3 STEPS TO HEALING AND WELLNESS

STEP 1. EMOTIONAL CHOICES
Take all memories, thoughts, feelings, and stresses out of the Unsafe Box and put them in the Safe Box.

STEP 2. NUTRITIONAL CHOICES
Eat a diet that is 75% alkaline ash, and 25% acid ash.

STEP 3. PHYSICAL CHOICES
Take a brisk 30 minute walk 5 days a week (or something comparable).

You will notice that each step has a word in common – the word *choices*. As adults, we make emotional, nutritional and physical *choices* that influence our health for good or bad. Our choices also greatly influence our children's ability to have good health and be well. They eat what we eat and largely follow the example we set in dealing with the physical and emotional aspects of life. As children get older and become teenagers, they become more and more responsible for their choices. Their health and wellness then eventually become their responsibility. Hopefully, they follow our good example, or at least return to it when their health gets bad.

Infants and younger children are either literally too young to make choices, or don't yet have the reasoning ability to make choices about what is good for their health. They are the main ones we want to talk about in this chapter. The younger children are, the more those decisions are made for them by their parents. When we talk about helping a child heal and become well, we often must talk to the parent.

Let's look at these Steps and see how they relate to children and what a parent can do to help his child be healthy and well. We will start with the easiest one first.

STEP 3. PHYSICAL CHOICES
Children need to exercise to be healthy just like adults. They do not need a regimented exercise plan. They just need to

be active. They need to go outside and play. Younger children tend to do this quite spontaneously. As they get older, they may need more encouragement to be involved. They need 30 minutes of exercise a day like adults. It may best found in organized athletics, dance classes, boy scouts, girl scouts, PE class, bicycling, and so on. As parents we need to encourage them to get off the couch or away from the computer or video game and to be involved.

STEP 2. NUTRITIONAL CHOICES

Let's start at the beginning. The ideal food for a newborn baby is, of course, mother's milk. Nothing can improve on that. An infant should consume its mother's milk exclusively until he or she is six months old, at which time other foods may begin to be added.

If a baby is having symptoms like colic, a runny nose, ear infections or skin conditions when drinking only mother's milk, then Mom needs to consider what she is eating or drinking as a cause. The milk she makes is affected by the food she eats. Too much meat, dairy, refined and processed foods, pop, tea and coffee can make her milk too toxic and too acid. She needs to alkalize and cleanse her body by eating vegetables and drinking lots of pure water until her baby's symptoms clear up, and then eat according to the diet discussed in Chapter 8. Fruits may be too cleansing at first, and make symptoms worse, so she should not add more of those until the baby's symptoms are gone. After the baby's symptoms have cleared she should slowly start adding fruits, always continuing with the vegetables.

The first regular foods to be introduced into a baby's diet should be fruits and vegetables. Mother's milk is an alkaline ash food and likewise so are most fruits and vegetables. In that sense, they are quite similar to mother's milk and ideal beginning foods. Fruits and vegetables also have a fairly short digestion time. This makes for an easier transition for the digestive tract as it adjusts to solid food. A few good fruits to begin with are a mashed banana, peach, pear or avocado. Some good vegetables to begin with are cooked squash, zucchini, carrots, sweet potatoes, or beets.

Whole grains, like breads, crackers and cereals, would be

the next food to add, but ideally not until the baby is one to two years old. Grains take longer to digest, and most leave an acid ash by-product. Digestive problems, diaper rash, other skin conditions and a runny nose can be good indicators too much grain has been eaten and the body is too acid, just as when mother's milk is too toxic. These symptoms are spill-over symptoms that result from the liver not being able to keep up with the amount of acid ash food consumed. Refined, processed flour and sugar products should not be consumed. Also be very aware of chemicals, flavor enhancers, and other food additives that can be very hard on young bodies and brains. Keep all food as whole and natural as possible.

Animal products such as meat and dairy should be the last foods introduced. These foods are acid forming and are not necessary to good health, but the body can handle them in limited quantities. Some may wonder whether or not their child needs cow's or goat's milk as he or she is weaned from mother's milk. This is a cultural consideration. Most children in the world are weaned to the food their parents eat and they drink water when thirsty. Dairy products are not necessary to good health. In my experience, dairy products are one of the major causes of childhood health problems. A runny nose, diaper rash, colic, ear infections, tonsillitis, skin rash, eczema, asthma, allergies, and even bed wetting are often caused by dairy products. We've seen the health of hundreds of children improve simply by quitting or cutting back on milk products.

By helping your children eat a diet that is 75 percent alkaline ash, you can assure the right nutritional choices are being made for their good health and well-being.

STEP 1. EMOTIONAL CHOICES

Children experience bad and stressful situations just as adults do. But they can't process them like an adult. They are innocent, and do not judge and reason the same way as an adult. So they cannot empty their Unsafe Box into their Safe Box in order to heal and be well. They don't have the conscious ability to do that.

At a young age, children are more like an animal in that they respond to their environment. A dog that is punished or corrected by its master will come to and seek comfort from that master. Small children punished or corrected by a parent will come to and seek comfort from that parent. As children get older, and begin to have a greater ability to judge and reason, they change and they will no longer automatically seek that parental comfort. We know then that they are no longer just responding to their environment but they are beginning to think things through for themselves.

Many pet owners will tell you their emotions are often reflected in their pets. If their dog is too aggressive, their cat too nervous, their parrot too troublesome or their horse too skittish, they look to themselves and their own feelings and actions to understand why. It is the same way with children. The younger they are, the more they will reflect the feelings they pick up from their parents, and especially their mother, the one to whom they are naturally the closest.

THE MOTHER-CHILD CONNECTION

Gail was easily able to comfort her eight month old grand-daughter, Randi. Yet, when she gave the baby back to her mother, the baby became fussy and irritable and started crying again. When Gail again took her grand-baby, once again she quickly calmed down.

Gail and her daughter soon realized that the stress Mom was under was being felt by baby Randi, and Mom needed to work on herself. Mom needed to identify and fix her own stress and get relaxed so her baby could relax. Sometimes we help our children the most by helping ourselves.

Stacey was surprised to learn how much her feelings literally affected her child. Her eighteen month old daughter, Jenny, had not gained any weight for two months. She'd had a chronic cough and a runny nose for over a year. Stacey was feeding her daughter really well, so nutrition was not likely the problem. Emotional stress had to be the answer.

I asked Stacey what was going on in her life when Jenny's problems began a year earlier (*Emotional Identifier #2 – When it Began*). Stacey remembered right away, because her whole family had been sick at the time. The washing machine in the apartment they were renting at the time was leaving rust spots on their clothes. After reporting it to the maintenance man, and then repeatedly confronting him about it, he reluctantly replaced it. The one he replaced it with smelled like mildew. The family all got sick after this replacement machine was brought into the apartment, and Stacey believed it was due to mold in the washer.

Now Stacey was in a dilemma. She didn't know what to do. How do you tell the maintenance man that you want another washing machine? She just couldn't get up the courage to confront him again, as he had not been pleasant to deal with the first time. Besides, they had bought a house and were moving several states away in a few months, and she thought they would just live with it until then.

Jenny had not been well since the washing machine episode. Stacey knew that is when her daughter got sick, and blamed the mold and especially herself for her daughter's poor health. Here is what Stacey said to me. Note the intensity of her feelings and where the blame is placed.

"I hate so much that she coughs like she does at night. I feel badly that it is my fault she has this problem because I couldn't stand up for myself and my family enough to tell the maintenance man that I didn't want him to leave the washing machine that smelled like mildew! If I could go back and just not make that service call, I would. I would just be grateful that the only problem we had was rust spots on our clothes. I would take a thousand rust spots over this!"

It is obvious that Stacey felt badly about this experience and was blaming herself for her daughter's health condition. I should note that Stacey was not without symptoms herself. Stacey had problems with dry hands, and they got really bad during this stressful situation. They cracked and bled and ac been very painful throughout the previous year.

I explained to Stacey that she had some letting go to do. She had stored this experience in a negative way in her Unsafe Box. Her negative feelings about it were not only keeping her from healing, but they were keeping Jenny from healing. Jenny was not old enough to have any idea of what was going on. But her *feeling* safe depended on her mother *feeling* safe. Like the dog reflecting his owner's feelings, Jenny was reflecting her mother's feelings.

This was a new way of looking at things for Stacey, but it made sense to her. We had treated her a few years earlier for a stressful situation. That one treatment had taken care of an ulcer and lactose intolerance she had suffered with for many years, so she was willing to try.

Within a week of gaining this new insight and doing some forgiving and letting go, both Stacey's hands and Jenny's coughing and runny nose had significantly improved. Then something happened. Their new house flooded. Stacey and her husband had bought a house eight months earlier, and now it had flooded – for the third time. The previous owners had said they had never had any water problems. Stacey and her husband had a hard time believing that and went to the realtor who sold the house to them to see what recourse they might have. The fear of confrontation was inevitable and Stacey's hands started to get worse, and so did Jenny.

Stacey was able to recognize the connection between the worsening of their symptoms and the confrontational feelings that were being stirred up again (*Emotional Identifier #1 – Current Stress*). As she fixed her reaction to the current stress and made it safe, a couple of similar earlier memories came to mind. She let go of them and put them in her Safe Box as well. A month later, this was Staceys's report, *"My hands are doing extremely well. I actually look now like I have thirty year old hands instead of ninety year old hands. It's beautiful. Jenny is also better by leaps and bounds. Her cough is all but gone, and her runny nose seems to have gone away as well. In the last six weeks she has gained two pounds, and is back up in the seventh percentile now instead of the first, where she was six weeks ago."*

Stacey had been reminded about what she needed to do to be healthy. She had also learned an important lesson about how to help her children be healthy. She concluded her thoughts to me by saying, *"The thought was new to me that Jenny could have such physical symptoms from feeling stress from me, and that by treating me, she could get better. I was a bit skeptical, but totally willing to try and it sure seems to have worked. So thanks!"*

SAFE FEELINGS

We have related many experiences of a person's symptoms beginning with something that happened early in life, before the age of reason. An experience is stored the way it is perceived at that early age. If it feels safe, it is safe; if it feels scary, it is scary. It is a fact. The idea to forgive or let go or brush off the experience does not enter young children's minds because they can't reason that way. The ability to choose to see it differently doesn't exist. It is easy to have an early childhood experience that "programs" us to be a certain way for the rest of our lives.

Parents have a role in assisting young children to program those experiences in a better way by helping them feel safe. The bad, unsafe experience can be made better by a parent who gives a hug, or comforts his child, or who listens and understands and explains. If the parent feels safe, then the child can feel safe. We've all seen the miracle of "kissing it better". Though parents can't fix everything, they can make a big difference. They can do something for the child the child can't do for himself. They can put the unsafe experience in the child's Safe Box *for* the child by offering love and comfort and a feeling that all is okay. What a blessing for the child! What a responsibility for the parents! When a child feels loved, safe, and protected, fear and worry of necessity must leave. The long-term beneficial effects are unlimited and immeasurable.

THE JUDGE'S SENTENCE

As parents we are responsible for our children and we generally know what is right and wrong and what is good and bad. We have goals and ideals for our children. We have a responsibility to train and teach them to not fight and quarrel but to love and serve, and other important principles.

A judge, in his courtroom, will issue a sentence. He can sentence a person to community service, to house arrest, or to prison. He can sentence the defendant to whatever he feels appropriate for the crime or behavior involved. That sentence can have a profound life-altering effect on the one receiving it.

As parents we may say words, or a sentence, that acts like

a *sentence* spoken by a judge. Consider the long term implications of children being given one of the following *sentences* by their "judge", even a loving judge.

> *"You're so dumb!"*
> *"Why can't you do anything right?"*
> *"You never listen!"*

Now consider the implications if they were given one of these sentences.

> *"You're so smart!"*
> *"You make such good choices!"*
> *"You always listen! Thank you!"*

Though we may think these sentences are just words, they can be much more powerful than that. They can literally *sentence* our children to a way of being. They may have the impact of an unalterable decree from a mighty judge. Those sentences can become part of their belief system, so they act accordingly, whether positive or negative. They can have a great impact on young children who accept them as facts, as they can't reason them otherwise. They can even have a great impact on a teenager or an adult. If asked, many adults can think of a statement to which they have been sentenced, and with thought, recognize its impact.

Melba grew up in a home where she was told she was different. She was different than her sister, and she often heard, *"Why are you so different?"* In her teens she acted out that being different by associating with those that were considered different. It was a self-destructive path with alcohol and drugs and all that goes with it.

Melba said she loved the theater because there she could act as if she was someone else. It gave her relief from being herself. Through high school and most of her working years, she dreaded night time and going to bed. It meant another day would follow, and she would have to go to school or work, where she was *different.*

At age sixty-two, Melba was diagnosed with Asperger's

Syndrome (a mild variation of Autism). Melba's health improved almost immediately and she began sleeping better than she had in many years after receiving this diagnosis. Why? Because she now knew *why* she was different. There was an explanation. She had spent most of her life questioning why she was different, and someone finally gave her the answer. It was Asperger's. She had a reason to be different, and she could now accept being different and live with that fact. Interestingly, her diagnosis was a Safe Box answer. It provided her relief and her health improved. Would Melba's life have been different if she had never heard the question, *"Why are you so different?"* Was Asperger's the *cause* of her being different, or was it a result of being told and believing that she was different?

A *sentence* may have a positive or a negative impact on us. Jonathon related that his former scout master had complimented him in a meeting and said that Jonathon was a person of integrity. He said Jonathon would always do what he said he would do. Jonathon said he didn't know for sure if that statement was true or if his scout master was just being nice, but it had a profound effect on him the rest of his life. He never forgot it. If he told someone he would do something, the memory of that comment was always in the back of his mind to make sure he would follow through.

Whether we are old or young, a *sentence* is a powerful thing. Since most of us are imperfect parents, we don't always say and do what we should. Thankfully a sentence may be annulled or changed, and another sentence be spoken in its place. *"I'm sorry." "It's my fault". "You are wonderful!" "Please forgive me."* Repentance is a wonderful gift and one that enables us to leave a positive *sentence* on our children.

As parents we have a great and wonderful opportunity to forever affect the lives of a few choice souls. Who knows for how many generations the effects of our lives will continue to be felt. The question is not one of whether or not we will affect our children's lives but one of *how*. Whether it is for good or bad, we make an impact. We need to be positive with them. We need to be their greatest source of strength and encouragement. No one else can do what we can for our own children. Our homes need to be a safe haven for them from the negative influences of the rest of the world.

In summary, the *3 Steps to Heal Yourself* apply to children just as much as to adults. They must be followed if we want our children to be healthy and well. We, as parents, have a vital and pivotal role in the application of these Steps.

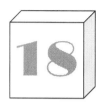

EMOTIONAL BAND-AIDS

You now better understand the cause of how we make ourselves sick, and what we can do to make ourselves well. So why don't we always apply it? The solution is often easier said than done. Living with an emotionally abusive spouse, or raising a handicapped child, or coping with a wayward teenager, or having financial problems, or having too many deadlines at work, or any one of a million other stresses can often be overwhelming. Sometimes, to help us in the process of healing, we need to use a Band-Aid.

COMFORT STRIPS

When your young son falls off his bike and skins his hands and knees, he immediately asks for a Band-Aid. Though these little plastic strips have no healing power, they are a comfort and they do help. Why is that? One reason is they help stop the bleeding. Another is they cushion and protect the wound from further injury and foreign particles while it heals. Could we apply something similar to a Band-Aid when our emotions have been injured or we are "stressed out"?

Martha was totally overwhelmed. She described herself as being completely dysfunctional. The stresses had been building in her life until one day she thought she would break.

The thing that saved Martha was a soothing music CD. As she listened she finally fell asleep and slept for three hours. When she awoke her perspective was brighter and she was gradually able to help herself back to normal living.

The CD did not do the healing. Healing comes from within. It did, though, help to emotionally "stop the bleeding" and "protect the wound" long enough for Martha to be able to regain emotional control. What are some of the Band-Aids available to us? There are as many Band-aids as there are people. As long as they allow us to escape or at least momentarily relieve the stress, they will have a positive comforting effect on the individual. Here is a list of some common Band-Aids.

Riding horses	Going for a walk	Walking the dog
Writing	Talking	Surfing the internet
Crocheting	Woodwork	Swimming
Chopping wood	Knitting	Texting
Bike riding	Cooking	Video games
Shopping	Reading	Medication
Counseling	Painting	Television
Puzzles	Eating	Meditation
Relaxation	Vacation	Music
Sleeping	Playing cards	Visualization
Work	Genealogy	Gardening

You will notice that these Band-Aids mainly work from the outside. They make the emotional injury or stress more tolerable. They distract us or allow us to escape from the thing that weighs on us. Though they may facilitate a quicker and easier healing, they also may occasionally prolong the cure. **The cure is always from the inside**. It is when we have a change of mind or a change of heart that the real healing of stress and hurts takes place.

DIRTY BAND-AIDS

Band-Aids are useful, but they can hinder the healing process if we are careless. A Band-Aid that is left on a sore too long can become dirty, and eventually infect the wound and make it worse. Its removal can sometimes even be a little painful. What is even worse is when we begin to believe that we can't heal without the help of a Band-Aid, or that we need a multiplicity of Band-Aids to get well. Several years ago we found our three year old son covered with twenty Band-Aids, necessary he felt, to heal all the mosquito bites he had.

Jane was having anxiety attacks. She knew they were stress related and she even knew what some of the problems were. She said, *"I worry about things that aren't likely to happen, like a car crash or a driving accident, but I can't help it. If I change what I am thinking to something more positive, I can often get rid of anxiety, but it doesn't last long. The negative thoughts soon come back, and the symptoms with them."*

Jane also said that as long as she was at home she was able to control her feelings quite well. When she went on a trip, the anxiety would become extremely bad. She would become extremely nervous, shake, sweat, get diarrhea, and develop severe headaches. The worst time was when she was on the verge of an "uncontrollable breakdown" in a foreign airport.

I asked Jane what she was doing for "Band-Aids". She said mainly controlling her thinking. That worked well at home, but not so well on a trip. To help that, her doctor prescribed a "Band-Aid" of medication for the last few trips she had taken, which had helped immensely. Now she was going on another trip and she had some new worries. *"What if the medication doesn't work this time? Maybe I am taking more than I should be. What if I get addicted to it? What about the side-effects?"* Her Band-Aids weren't working well for her anymore. She couldn't control her thinking and was uncertain of her medication, and so now she had come to see me. Why? She was in search of another, more powerful Band-Aid. She was still trying to resolve her anxiety attacks from the outside.

We can see how Jane's Band-Aids had helped her handle her stress. As long as she could control her thinking, she felt fine. The medication had also calmed her. We can also see how she had thought they were the instruments of healing. Just like a dirty Band-Aid, they were beginning to infect the wound and compound the problem. She was finding that she could not always control her thinking and the fear of the side effects of the medication was becoming stronger than its benefits. They needed to be removed and replaced with a new, clean Band-Aid. More importantly, Jane needed to learn that the true healing comes from the inside, and that the Band-Aid is only a temporary help.

What was it that Jane needed to change inside? She is no different than the rest of us. She needed to let go of fear and replace it with faith. As long as she was in control, she was fine. As long as she was in control, there was less anxiety and that is why home was so much more comfortable to her. When she traveled, however, there were too many things out of her control, and that produced fear as she imagined the hundreds of things that could go wrong. The solution to her anxiety was to identify and deal with the cause and give control to Heavenly Father and trust His will to be done. When a *"What if..."* thought came, she needed to immediately replace it with *"Thy will be done!"* in order to remind herself of who was in charge. Though she did have faith, it was conditional. She had been trusting in Heavenly Father as long as things turned out the way she wanted. When they didn't, or it didn't appear they would, she wanted to immediately retake control.

Taking this big step for Jane was difficult. She had relied on her Band-Aids in the past and had given them the credit for controlling her anxiety. Removing the old Band-Aids, exposing the wound so to speak, and allowing healing from the inside was painful and fearful. Those "plastic strips" of control had been there a long time and had adhered securely. But it was a necessary step for her to truly become well. The results of Jane's efforts in turning control over to God were remarkable. She felt more relaxed and more at peace than she had in a long time. That's not to say she didn't struggle in her efforts to give up control. It took time and much prayer and scripture reading, but she was able to do it and her life and health were better because of it.

FAVORITE BAND-AIDS

To help her through the healing process, I gave Jane another Band-Aid to use, with the explanation that it was only temporary. It's a favorite Band-Aid I like to give patients to use as I feel it does more than most to encourage healing from the inside. It's the following simple little assignment.

Think a thousand thankful thoughts a day!

Why does this work? For one thing, it's a catchy little phrase so it is easy to remember. But the main reason is that it takes a lot of time to think a thousand thankful thoughts. When you are thinking a thankful thoughts you cannot think a negative thought. The two cannot be in your mind at the same time anymore than light and darkness can be in the same place at the same time. Fear cannot exist, or any other negative thought, which enables your mind and body to heal.

Another reason this simple little exercise works is because you can think a thousand thankful thoughts anywhere, doing anything, even in the midst of your greatest stress. A Band-Aid such as riding a horse or crocheting would not be so appropriate or convenient.

Another favorite Band-Aid I recommend is singing. *"Music hath charms to soothe a savage breast, to soften rocks, or bend a knotted oak,"* said William Congreve, a seventeenth century poet. (www.bartleby.com/100/212.1.html).

I'm not sure about it softening rocks, but it definitely softens the soul and brings a person a sense of peace. Singing, listening, and creating music of any kind will provide an immediate biological and psychological benefit. That must be why people sing in the shower and while driving the car, or simply listen to music that's inspiring and distracting from emotional upset.

I learned this lesson when I was a teenager, and I never forgot it. It has been a great benefit to me. A friend, Ross, reported that singing hymns the two miles from work to home allowed him to leave all his stress at work, and be ready to enjoy his family when he arrived.

IF A LITTLE IS GOOD, IS MORE BETTER?

If we look back at the sample list of Band-Aids, we see that they can all be done to excess. That may only result in a waste of time, or it could result in bad habits and even addictions. Some of the more negative Band-Aids, such as tobacco, alcohol, drugs and pornography we have not even mentioned. They can be extremely destructive.

Here is a good exercise to do.

Make a list of the five Band-Aids you use the most to overcome the effects of stress. (This may require some introspection in order to recognize them.) They may or may not be included in the list we previously described.

1. _____
2. _____
3. _____
4. _____
5. _____

Now analyze each one of these five Band-Aids. Are any of them being done in excess? Are they leading to a waste of time, bad habits, addictions, or even self-destruction? Do they need to be changed, or replaced? The ideal change to make is to replace your fears with faith and deal with their cause. However, Band-Aids are permissible and even necessary at times, and we all can benefit from the comfort and protection they give.

If you need to, make another list of Band-Aids to turn to in times of stress, replacing the ones that are inappropriate. Make them ones you enjoy, that are comforting to you, and yet are easy to control. You might consider using singing a song or thinking a thousand thankful thoughts since they are very powerful and positive Band-Aids.

1. _____
2. _____
3. _____
4. _____
5. _____

You should now be well equipped to handle any stress that comes your way. With faith and a few Band-Aids you can overcome any challenge you may face.

CONCLUSION

The body is the most marvelous creation on earth. It always does what it is told. It is a wonderful instrument that does everything it does for a reason. As we give it good quality food and drink, adequate exercise, and keep it physically and emotionally safe, it will reward us with health, vitality and energy throughout our entire lives.

We now understand how we can interfere with the body's automatic processes and make ourselves sick. We also know the 3 steps to healing and wellness. I will repeat them once again.

3 STEPS TO HEALING AND WELLNESS

STEP 1. EMOTIONAL CHOICES
Take all memories, thoughts, feelings, and stresses out of the Unsafe Box and put them in the Safe Box.

STEP 2. NUTRITIONAL CHOICES
Eat a diet that is 75% alkaline ash, and 25% acid ash.

STEP 3. PHYSICAL CHOICES
Take a brisk 30 minute walk 5 days a week (or something comparable).

I have seen thousands of patients apply these 3 steps to regain their health and be well.

WHAT IF I'M STUCK?

As you implement the *3 Steps to Heal Yourself* your health and vitality always improve. However you may also reach a point where you are stuck, where you still have pain or another symptom that fails to get better. What do you do then?

There are really two answers:

1. Gain and apply more knowledge.
2. Ask for help.

As you seek more knowledge and ask for help, remember to always relate it to the foundational principles of health we have discussed – the body is doing what it is doing for a reason and that there are only three causes of the symptoms you have.

My intent in writing this book has been to empower you to heal yourself. I believe with all my heart you have that ability. I know you can do it if you apply the principles we have discussed.

There is much more information we could share with you that is impossible to put in a book this size. Much of that is available for free at www.3stepstohealyourself.com. Click on the *Help Yourself* section to watch free classes, videos and workshops and to download free articles and other information. This area will frequently be updated so you will want to check it often. The information is all placed there to help you heal yourself. You will need to enter your email address to access this section.

You may also want to visit our Wilde Natural Health Center FaceBook Page as we often post natural health news, tips and suggestions there.

The second key to getting "unstuck" is to ask for help. Sometimes we need someone with a different perspective or outlook to help us see what we are doing to ourselves.

Marsha had two problems, a wrist she had hurt six months earlier and a leg that was swelling. She had been to the doctor and was told she would likely need surgery on her wrist and a compression stocking for her leg. She had tried applying the principles we teach and only improved slightly.

As we talked to Marsha about the possible things causing her symptoms, she was able to see things differently. In five days her wrist pain was gone and the swelling had left her leg.

If you are stuck in your progress and are in need of help like Marsha, call our office and ask for the *Heal Yourself Consultation.* This is a free telephone consultation I am offering exclusively to readers of *The Safe Box of Health.*

You can set up an appointment with my staff or leave a message and we will call you back. The telephone number is 1-866-DrWilde (1-866-379-4533). Please be patient with us as we get back to you. As the author of this book, and a believer in its principles, it is important to me that you are able to heal yourself. So if you are stuck and need help, please call and allow us to help you individually with your health.

I conclude with the story of Tess.

Tess was fifty-six years old and had had constant back pain for five years. She had chronic pain in her right knee, even though she'd had surgery on it twice. She had a difficult time sleeping because of the pain she was in. Tess applied the 3 Steps to Healing and Wellness and in two months was pain free and able to sleep through the night.

Like most patients we treat with chronic symptoms, Tess had to improve her diet. She needed to eat many more fruits and vegetables and drink more water. She especially needed to learn how to better deal with stress and let go of undesirable things that had happened to her in her life.

Tess was very busy and overwhelmed with all the things she had to do. She and her husband were building a house. She was a waitress. She trimmed horses' hooves and did horse massage. By the end of a typical day she could hardly move because of pain. She finally had to admit to herself that she had "too many irons in the fire" and she couldn't possibly keep up with all that needed to be done. She quit her waitressing job which helped greatly to relieve the stress of too much to do and allow her to better manage her time.

Tess also used several of the *Emotional Identifiers* to understand how her reactions to past experiences were contributing to the symptoms she was having. Her back pain started five years earlier when she moved from Washington to Minnesota. She had blamed the back pain on the move, but as she reflected more closely on what was happening at that time, she realized the cause. Tess had been divorced and had remarried and was moving to Minnesota with her new husband. The move meant leaving her fifteen year old daughter in Washington. The "weight" of that decision and how it had impacted her daughter had never left her, and was a major cause of the constant back pain she had. In the process of letting that go, she called and talked to her daughter about that decision. They had a wonderful visit, and it was a very healing conversation.

Tess' mother had passed away seven years earlier, and Tess couldn't think about that without feeling sad and having tears come to her eyes. She realized that this memory was also weighing on her. She and her mother had always been "out of sorts" with each other, and Tess had been raised mainly by her grandparents.

One memory was particularly poignant and helped Tess let go of unresolved feelings toward her mother. When Tess was five she was bitten by the neighbor's pet coyote and ended up in the hospital. She said, *"As I lay in the hospital, my mother was no where to be found."* Tess realized that she had felt abandoned by her mother, and that this experience had been repeated in several other situations as she matured. She worked on these and other memories, and made them safe. As a result, her pain disappeared and she was able to sleep all night long. Tess commented, *"I have learned to see negative things as simply a challenge to overcome, and that with God's help I can do it."*

Tess, like many others, had learned that she was in charge of her health and could literally heal herself.

I hope you have been inspired by this book. I hope it has opened your eyes to what you can do to have a lifetime of health and wellness. As you implement these *3 Steps to Heal Yourself*, improved health is an automatic and natural outcome. You can have your own special experience as you heal and your health improves. You can then write your own story, *I Healed Myself.*

For more information, videos, downloads, classes and workshops, go to the *Help Yourself* section at:

www.3stepstohealyourself.com

For a **FREE** personal *Heal Yourself Consultation,* exclusive to readers of *The Safe Box of Health,* call:

1-866DrWilde (1-866-379-4533)

7567578R0

Made in the USA
Charleston, SC
18 March 2011